5G Wireless Communication System in Healthcare Informatics

This text discusses problems and needs with the implementation of a 5G mobile communications system in the healthcare sector. It covers the issues related to advanced modulation schemes, telehealth, and remote diagnosis. It discusses important topics including virtual healthcare monitoring, spectrum sensing techniques, the role of 5G in medical applications, the role of nano-communication in healthcare informatics, and remote diagnosis. The text will be useful for graduate students, academic researchers, and professionals in the fields of electrical, and electronics and communication engineering, and allied healthcare.

This book;

- Discusses novel architecture to manage the allocation of resources, and the interference issue among existing and advanced radios
- Provides focus to estimate the performance, cost and accommodation of the next generation technology design for the IoT, modern health- care, and education
- Covers advanced technologies and their role in healthcare
- Discusses key topics including spectrum access, advanced waveforms, which can help in standardization of 5G based smart hospital
- Explores the impact of telemedicine in smart healthcare.

This reference text covers the latest advances in the field of 5G mobile communication for healthcare informatics, addressing both original algorithm development and new applications of 5G mobile Communications.

Advances in Antenna Design, Wireless Communication and Mobile Network Technology Series
Edited by Manoj Gupta, Ghanshyam Singh and Pradeep Kumar

5G Wireless Communication System in Healthcare Informatics
Manoj Gupta, Arun Kumar, Basant Agarwal, Korhan Cengiz and Ghanshyam Singh

5G Wireless Communication System in Healthcare Informatics

Edited by
Manoj Gupta, Arun Kumar,
Basant Agarwal, Korhan Cengiz, and
Ghanshyam Singh

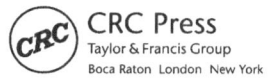

CRC Press
Taylor & Francis Group
Boca Raton London New York

CRC Press is an imprint of the
Taylor & Francis Group, an **informa** business

First edition published 2023
by CRC Press
6000 Broken Sound Parkway NW, Suite 300, Boca Raton, FL 33487-2742

and by CRC Press
4 Park Square, Milton Park, Abingdon, Oxon, OX14 4RN

CRC Press is an imprint of Taylor & Francis Group, LLC

ISBN: 9781032312194 (hbk)
ISBN: 9781032436593 (pbk)
ISBN: 9781003368311 (ebk)

DOI: 10.1201/9781003368311

Typeset in Times
by Newgen Publishing UK

Contents

Preface

The Role of 5G Communication and Healthcare Informatics is an emerging field of research at the intersection of information science, computer science, mobile communication systems, digital health and healthcare informatics. Healthcare informatics and analytics is a new era that brings tremendous opportunities and challenges due to plenty of easily available medical data for further analysis. The aim of wireless communication in healthcare informatics is to ensure high-quality, efficient healthcare, better treatment, and quality of life by efficiently analyzing abundant medical and healthcare data, including patient's data, electronic health records and lifestyle. This book provides comprehensive details on 5G applications and effectiveness, ensuring a high spectral efficiency, accurate detection and latency <1 ms. It is also concluded that the 5G network helps in the expansion of healthcare by developing a modern smart hospital backed by 5G networks.

The book will play a vital role in improving human life to a great extent. Any researchers and practitioners will benefit highly, especially those working in the fields of mobile communication systems, digital health, intelligent medicine and health informatics. This book is a good collection of state-of-the-art approaches for 5G communication systems-based medical and healthcare related applications. It will be very beneficial for new researchers and practitioners working in the field to quickly understand the best performing methods. They would be able to compare different approaches and can carry forward their research in this most important area of research which has a direct impact on betterment of human life and health. This book will be very useful because there is no book on the market that provides a good collection of state-of-the-art methods of advances in 5G communication systems for medical and health informatics since the role of mobile communications has recently emerged and is a very new field of research in medical and healthcare informatics.

It describes needs, problems in the implementation of the 5G mobile communication system in the healthcare sector. It also covers the issues related to advanced modulation schemes, telehealth, and remote diagnosis. This book will assist researchers, academicians and students pursuing courses of medical electronics as well as the impact of 5G wireless communications in healthcare informatics.

Chapter 1 presents a brief survey about 5G in healthcare. In this chapter, the authors provide a brief overview of the 5G network with specific applications to healthcare along with its advantages and disadvantages. Further, authors introduced the concept of smart healthcare and the focus towards artificial intelligence providing solutions to many computational challenges and efficient resource allocation. 5G technology would revolutionize the way we use healthcare services and would lead to better and fair allocation of healthcare services in society.

Chapter 2 covers advances of 5G wireless communication systems in healthcare informatics. The healthcare sector is a very important aspect of the 5G communication system. H-IoT will play a very important function in shaping the future of human beings in healthcare 5.0. A 5G communication system with BSN will lead to personalized well-being in future. The various communication layers and the corresponding technologies help us to understand the H-IoT. The H-IoT faces various security challenges. The solutions of these security issues are proposed by various researchers. Numerous communication protocols are proposed in application, service, and in the infrastructure of H-IoT. The use of H-IoT devices and diagnostic tools will increase in the future very rapidly. H-IoT is an integral part of the 5G communication network.

Chapter 3 covers beamforming in massive MIMO communications for 5G technology. In this chapter, authors provide a tutorial of modeling and analyzing significant key performance indicators (KPIs) of massive multi-input multi-output (MIMO) systems in a downlink Rayleigh fading channel.

Chapter 4 covers 5G-enabled network technology trends for smart healthcare systems. The chapter provides a comprehensive analysis of 5G-supported smart healthcare solutions on the IoT. By classifying existing literature, a framework for 5G smart healthcare is proposed. Finally, with the IoT and 5G smart healthcare solution, this chapter address many open problems and study challenges.

Chapter 5 covers practical considerations relating to non-orthogonal multiple access transmission for 5G technology. It deals with investigating practical NOMA transmission using a variety of approaches. First, authors constructed PD-NOMA using AWGN and Rayleigh channels, and then they used ZF to decode the data. Then they developed CD-NOMA, decoding using SCMA and extracting data from users with MPA. Finally, they implemented a realistic transmission scenario in which users were randomly assigned to cells and a downlink network with a single base station servicing a group of users was employed. The system demonstrates that not all possible NOMA users are regarded as NOMA users. Additionally, authors created a downlink PD-NOMA in NOMA users and displayed the BER performance as well as the sum rate of NOMA users.

Chapter 6 covers comparisons of UTD-PO and FKE models for path loss prediction over an irregular terrain. In this paper, authors have proposed a comparative study for the path loss prediction of mobile radio waves over an irregular terrain scenario based on a uniform theory of diffraction–physical optics (UTD-PO) and Fresnel-Kirchhoff knife edge diffraction theory (FKE). The comparative results show that when the number of obstacles increases in the terrain between the point of transmission and the points of reception, the predicted path loss of the FKE approach gives inferior results in comparison to the path loss of the measurement data and the predicted path loss of the UTD-PO approach. Also, the data analysis of these approaches shows that the mean error of path loss obtained for the UTD-PO approach is smaller in comparison to the mean error of path loss for the FKE approach.

Chapter 7 covers integrated blockchain and MEC systems empowered healthcare services. In this chapter, authors present the possible integration between healthcare IoT devices, MEC, blockchain, and AI as a base for future healthcare systems. Authors also explore the latest state, the shortcomings and the research opportunities of this integration.

Chapter 8 covers optimized cognitive radio networks for 5G technology. In this work, authors propose an optimum beamforming design using the genetic algorithm with multi-parent crossover (GA-MPC), and cross-entropy (CE) to improve the performance of the energy detector-based spectrum sensing method.

Chapter 9 covers gamified wearables in childhood obesity therapy driven by 5G wireless communication systems with special emphasis on Pacific Island Countries. Compared to the traditional methods, gamification has shown a new alternative model for healthcare. Due to the widespread use of mobile phones, laptops, and the like, the potential to use gamification in the control and prevention of obesity is enormous. With the increase in 5G network coverage the potential to use gamification increases many times. The mobile applications can not only be used to deliver health-related messages and physical activity components of any of the programs but can also be used to collect, compile, analyze and access the data easily at the click of the button. This chapter contains an overview of the literature and the design of the qualitative study conducted in Pacific Island countries. This chapter also summarizes various interventions that used gamified wearables conducted in these countries and the major limitations identified by these studies. It also highlights the recommendations given by researchers. In brief, these recommendations are realistic methods for obesity management, enticing game strategy, challenging incentives, and constructive education.

Chapter 10 covers the role of photonics in the realization of future 6G communication systems. This chapter discusses the key enabling technologies of 6G communication systems and the importance of photonics in realizing these 6G technologies. This chapter also presents the recent development of photonics for 6G communication.

Chapter 11 covers the MIMO antenna for IoT and ISM band applications. In this chapter, authors describe a design of antenna that achieves specific important requirements. 5G communications are likely to include MIMO, which will necessitate antennas with a large number of elements. However, maintaining strong isolation between ports is difficult due to the size constraint. With the use of HFSS software, authors built a MIMO antenna having improved isolation. An efficient four-element mm-wave MIMO (multiple-input multiple-output) antenna is being proposed for use in a 5G system.

Chapter 12 covers the role of Terahertz photoconductive antennas in future healthcare informatics. In this chapter, THz generation and detection using various methods, starting from electrical, optical, and electro-optic methods has been described. However, the focus is given to PCA as it is the best possible way of THz generation and detection. For PCA, the classifications, equivalent circuital analysis, numerical simulations, and experimental characterization has been reported in detail.

Acknowledgment

Our efforts to produce a book in the evolving field of Advances of 5G Wireless Communication Systems in healthcare Informatics culminate efforts from several scientists, academicians, and practitioners across the world. The invited call for contributions in this fast-growing and rapidly evolving field has received an overwhelming response from the fraternity around the globe. A total of 44 proposals have been received for this book. Each of these proposal manuscripts has been thoroughly checked and peer reviewed by at least three reviewers who are renowned experts in the respective topic. Based on the peer review outcomes and the suitability of the revised manuscript on the book's theme, 12 high-quality works have been chosen for final publication. We express our sincere thanks to all our reviewers for sparing their valuable time and sharing their expertise. We also express our sincere gratitude and best wishes to all the authors for contributing quality research work related to the book. We are also thankful to the New Horizon College of Engineering, Bengaluru (India), Indian Institute of Information Technology Kota (India), Malviya National Institute of Technology Jaipur (India) and Trakya University Turkey for extending their support in every way possible for this book. Finally, we are also very thankful to the publishers' team of CRC press for their support at every stage, which helped us in the timely production of this book. We hope that this book will be handy for students and expert researchers working in the relevant domains.

Editors

Manoj Gupta earned his Ph.D. from the University of Rajasthan, Jaipur (India). He earned his M.Tech in Digital Signal Processing from H.N.B Garhwal Central University, Uttarakhand, India and B.Tech degree in Electronics and Communication Engineering from the Institute of Engineering and Technology, M. J. P. Rohilkhand University Campus, Bareilly (U.P.) India. His overall experience is more than 15 years. He has published many research papers in international journals and National/International conferences. He has been granted two patents and two Indian Research Copyrights and published 5 Patents to his credit. His research interests are in biomedical signal and image processing, soft computing, computational intelligence, biomedical engineering, artificial intelligence and antenna and wireless communication systems. He is a member of many professional bodies such as the IEEE, IACSIT, ISTE, IAENG and many more. He has served as technical programme committee (TPC) member and reviewer in various international conferences such as, ICCIA 2020, ICCIA 2019 ICSIP 2018, ICSIP 2017, ICSIP 2016, AIPR 2017, AIPR 2016, ICCIA 2018, ICCIA 2017, ICCIA 2016, ICNIT 2018 and many more. He was invited to be keynote speaker/invited speaker in 2017 2nd IEEE International Conference on Signal and Image Processing (ICSIP 2017), August 04–06, 2017 in Nanyang Executive Centre, Singapore and Invited for Keynote Speaker in 2017 International Conferences on Public Health and Medical Sciences (ICPHMS 2017), May 23–24, 2017 in Xi'an, China. He is associate editor and reviewer of many international journals. His name has been listed in Marquis Who's Who in Science and Engineering® USA in 2012, 2016 and Marquis Who's Who in the World® USA in 2010 (28th Edition), 2011 (29th edition) and 2013 (31st edition).

Arun Kumar earned his Ph.D. in electronics and communication engineering from JECRC University, Jaipur, India. He is an Associate Professor in Electronics and Communication Engineering at New Horizon College of Engineering in Bengaluru, India. Dr. Kumar has a total of 8.5 years of teaching experience and has published more than 75 research articles in SCI-E and Scopus Index journals. His research interests are advanced waveforms for 5G mobile communication systems and 5G-based smart hospitals, PAPR reduction techniques in the multicarrier waveform, and spectrum sensing techniques. Dr. Kumar has successfully implemented different reduction techniques for multi-carrier waveforms such as NOMA, FBMC, UFMC, and so on, and has also implemented and compared different waveform techniques for the 5G system. Currently, he is working on the requirements of a 5G-based smart hospital system. He is a member of the IEEE and a reviewer for many refereed, indexed journals.

Basant Agarwal is an assistant professor at the Indian Institute of Information Technology Kota (IIIT-Kota), India. He earned a Ph.D. and M.Tech. from the Department of CSE, MNIT Jaipur. He has worked as a postdoctoral research fellow at the Norwegian University of Science and Technology (NTNU), Norway, under the prestigious ERCIM (European Research Consortium for Informatics and Mathematics) fellowship in 2016. He has also worked as a research scientist at Temasek Laboratories, National University of Singapore (NUS), Singapore. He has published more than 60 reputed conferences and Journals. Dr. Agarwal is serving as a senior member, technical program committee member, member of the editorial boards/reviewer boards of various renowned international conferences/journals such as knowledge-based Systems, IEEE intelligent systems, information processing and management to name but a few. His research interest is in artificial intelligence, text mining, natural language processing, machine learning, deep learning, intelligent systems, expert systems and related areas.

Korhan Cengiz earned a B.S. degree in electronics and communication engineering from Kocaeli University, Kocaeli, Turkey, in 2008, an M.S. degree in electronics and communication engineering from Namik Kemal University, Tekirdag, Turkey, in 2011, and a Ph.D. degree in electronics engineering from Kadir Has University, Istanbul, Turkey, in 2016. From 2009 to 2013, he was a research assistant at the Department of Telecommunications, Namik Kemal University. From 2013 to 2018, he was a lecturer at the Department of Telecommunications, Trakya University. Since 2018, he has been an assistant professor with the Electrical-Electronics Engineering Department, Trakya University, Edirne, Turkey. He is the author of over 30 articles. His research interests include wireless sensor networks, routing protocols, wireless communications, statistical signal processing, indoor positioning systems, power electronics and 5G. He is an editor of the Turkish Journal of Electrical *Engineering and Computer Sciences*. Dr. Cengiz's awards and honors include the Tubitak Priority Areas Ph.D. Scholarship and the Kadir Has University Ph.D. Student Scholarship.

Ghanshyam Singh is a full professor with the Department of Electronics and Communication Engineering, Malaviya National Institute of Technology (MNIT) Jaipur, India. He worked as a visiting research scholar/professor at HW University Edinburgh (UK), UEF Joensuu (Finland) and Keio University (Japan). He has published over 150 research articles in peer reviewed journals and conferences. He is a senior member of SPIE, OSA, IEEE and a Fellow of OSI and IETE. He is the recipient of the 2017 IEEE Distinguished Lecturer Award of the Photonics Society. In the past, he had joint research collaborations with the researchers from Keio University (Japan), University of Vienna (Austria), LNPU (Ukraine) and Cairo University (Egypt). He is presently collaborating on a multi-institutional project with researchers from University of KwaZulu-Natal (South Africa), PSUTI Samara (Russia) and USTC Shanghai (China) for a BRICS STI Framework Program. His current research interest includes micro and nano-structured photonic devices for integrated photonics, nano-structured materials, quantum photonics, photonic crystal fibers, and so forth.

Contributors

Basant Agarwal
Indian Institute of Information
  Technology Kota
Kota, Rajasthan, India

Asmaa U. Al-Saggaf
King Abdulaziz University
Jeddah, Saudi Arabia.

Ubaid M. Al-Saggaf
King Abdulaziz University
Jeddah, Saudi Arabia

Abdulah Aljohani
King Abdulaziz University
Jeddah, Saudi Arabia

Ibrahim Almujtaba
King Abdulaziz University
Jeddah, Saudi Arabia

Mohammed Ali Ahmed Alrefaei
King Abdulaziz University
Jeddah, Saudi Arabia.

Abdulrahman U. Alsaggaf
King Abdulaziz University
Jeddah, Saudi Arabia

Amira A. Amer
Cairo University
Giza, Egypt

Yash Bhardwaj
M.J.P Rohilkhand University,
Bareilly, Uttar Pradesh, India

E. Nisha Flora Boby
SRM Institute of Science and
  Technology,
Chennai, Tamilnadu, India

Kamal Kishor Choure
Malaviya National Institute of
  Technology,
Jaipur, Rajasthan

Jitendra Kumar Deegwal
Government Women Engineering
  College
Ajmer, Rajasthan, India

Ahmad Kamal Hassan
Ghulam Ishaq Khan Institute of
  Engineering Sciences and Technology
Topi, Khyber Pakhtunkhwa, Pakistan

Tawfik Ismail
Cairo University
Giza, Egypt

Sandeep Joshi
Birla Institute of Technology &
  Science (BITS)
Pilani, Rajasthan, India

Inderpreet Kaur
M.J.P Rohilkhand University,
Bareilly, Uttar Pradesh, India

Ashok Kumar
Government Women Engineering
  College
Ajmer, Rajasthan, India

D. K. Lobiyal
Jawaharlal Nehru University
New Delhi, New Delhi, India

Muhammad Moinuddin
King Abdulaziz University
Jeddah, Saudi Arabia

Shyamal Mondal
Defense Institute of Advance
  Technology
Pune, Maharashtra, India

Nitesh Mudgal
Poornima College of Engineering
Jaipur, Rajasthan, India

Rahul Mukherjee
Bennett University
Greater Noida, Uttar Pradesh, India

Manisha Prajapat
Malaviya National Institute of
  Technology,
Jaipur, Rajasthan

Puspa Devi Pukhrambam
National Institute of Technology Silchar
Silchar, Assam, India

Rashmi
Jaipur National University
Jaipur, Rajasthan, India

Vaisshale Rathinasamy
Amrita School of Engineering, Amrita
  Vishwa Vidyapeetham
Chennai, Tamilnadu, India

Ankur Saharia
Manipal University Jaipur
Jaipur, Rajasthan, India

Yashu Shanker
Jawaharlal Nehru University
New Delhi, New Delhi, India

Sanjeev Sharma
R.D. Engineering College
Ghaziabad, Uttar Pradesh, India

Ghanshyam Singh
Malaviya National Institute of
  Technology
Jaipur, Rajasthan, India

Hari Kumar Singh
M.J.P Rohilkhand University
Bareilly, Uttar Pradesh, India

Navneet Singh
M.J.P Rohilkhand University, Bareilly
Bareilly, Uttar Pradesh, India

Pragya Singh
Fiji National University, Fiji
Suva, Fiji, Fiji Island

Satyanand Singh
Fiji National University
Suva, Fiji, Fiji Island

Manish Tiwari
Manipal University Jaipur
Jaipur, Rajasthan, India

Vinita Tiwari
Indian Institute of Information
  Technology Kota
Kota, Rajasthan, India

Harpreet Vohra
Thapar Institute of Engineering and
  Technology
Patiala, Punjab, India

Ajay Yadav
Bennett University,
Greater Noida, Uttar Pradesh, India

1 5G in Healthcare
A Survey

Sandeep Joshi, Vinita Tiwari, and Basant Agarwal

CONTENTS

1.1 INTRODUCTION

The advent of fifth generation (5G) and beyond 5G (B5G) communications has opened vast areas of application including automation and prediction in various fields, prominently in healthcare. 5G is described as a next generation communication technology which can support higher data rates, provide ultra-low latency with reliable communication, and which has many other advantages as shown in Table 1.1 which gives a comparison of 5G characteristics in comparison to previous generation communication technology, that is, fourth generation (4G). Applications of 5G in healthcare would transform the healthcare industry, changing the way various services such as patient services, treatment, wellness programs, consultations, and surgeries are performed. The ultra-fast, highly efficient, ultra-reliable, and massive machine connectivity of a 5G network will help the healthcare services to reach every user. 5G opens new opportunities in healthcare [2], specifically:

a) *telehealth*: which allows patients to get medical care from the comfort of their homes, which according to market research [2], would have a growth rate of 16.5% over the period 2017–2023,
b) *large medical files transfer:* 5G would allow the instant transfer of medical imagery files which are large files needing large amounts of data. Each patient generates hundreds of gigabytes of data and in total the healthcare industry generates massive amounts of data and thus, the need for a technology that supports such high bandwidth and data rates,

DOI: 10.1201/9781003368311-1

TABLE 1.1
A Comparison of 5G and 4G Characteristics

Characteristics	4G	5G
Latency	30 – 50 ms	1 – 10 ms
Throughput	300 Mbps – 1 Gbps	10 Gbps
User data rates	20 – 50 Mbps	Up to 1 Gbps
Connected devices per unit area	12	100

Source: [1].

c) *real time monitoring:* remote real time monitoring can be done with the support of 5G wearable devices transferring real time data over the 5G network. A report by Accenture [2], claims that this real time monitoring would reduce hospital costs by 16% over the next five years, and

d) *medical innovation:* real time monitoring would need effective sensors to capture correct data and reliable transmission over the network, this would fuel innovation in the design of medical sensors that are expected to be low-cost and efficient.

The telecom industry is an important partner to the healthcare industry with an important role to play in the smart healthcare industry, finding applications in different healthcare categories as described below [3].

a) *patient applications:* precision medicine and monitoring,

b) *hospital applications:* telemetry and virtual reality in surgery procedures, and

c) *data management:* medical data record maintenance and delivery.

Healthcare centers would turn into data centers and 5G technology would help in making sense out of the data which would include techniques such as artificial intelligence (AI) in processing the data.

Telehealth and remote home monitoring technology have the potential to resolve the issues of healthcare in rural areas with doctors located miles away. According to a study by Market Research Future, the telemedicine market is expected to grow at a compound annual growth rate of 16.5% from 2017 to 2023. The study determined that the reason for the predicted increase is demand in rural areas for healthcare, as well as a rise in government initiatives for people in rural areas, with doctors located several miles away. However, medical images generally use very large file sizes which need high bandwidth and thus causes an additional burden on the existing network, resulting in congestion. 5G technology has potential to overcome this issue with high data rates, low latency, and high bandwidth and durability per unit area [1].

5G wireless embraces a heterogeneous set of integrated air interfaces and relies on new technologies, namely, mobile edge computing, fog computing, software defined

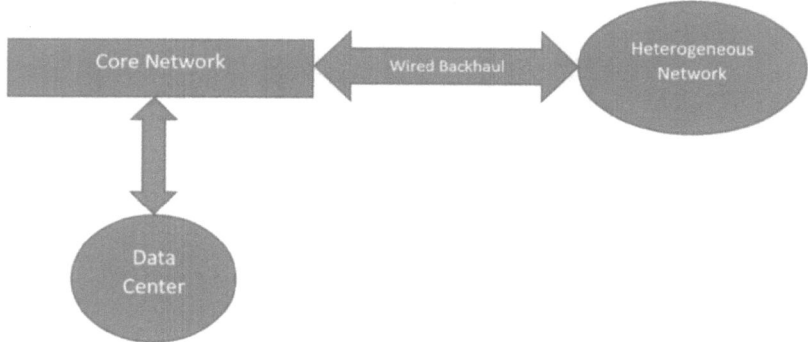

FIGURE 1.1 A generic 5G communication network based architecture for healthcare applications. (Adapted from [5, 6].)

radio, device-to-device (D2D) communications, and the like, to achieve high performance, scalability, and intelligence.

5G promises to provide ultra-reliable services and transform the user–centric network to a massive machine–centric network by enabling billions of devices. Basically, 5G is much more than simply a next generation technology, it is much more transformative. 5G networks combine cellular and satellite solutions to offer a high level of flexibility and a uniform spectrum for a wide range of frequencies ranging from lower GHz to millimeter waves and beyond.

1.2 5G ARCHITECTURE AND KEY TECHNOLOGIES FOR HEALTHCARE

5G technology is envisaged to provide high data rates and ultra-low latency which opens up applications in many areas of interest to human beings, one important area finding variety of applications is healthcare [4–8]. Latency plays an important role in healthcare applications such as robotic surgery and is critical in applications involving remote surgery. The generic architecture of the 5G network is as depicted in Figure 1.1, in which the interaction between the core and the heterogeneous network is shown. The 5G core network will be connected to the data center on one side and to the heterogeneous network on the other side. The connection with the heterogeneous network will be through wired backhaul supporting higher data rates and thus, providing greater flexibility. Figure 1.2 shows a suggested application of robotic surgery in a generic 5G communication based network. The key aspects expected of the network for such applications are latency of 25 ms or lower, failure rate of approximately 10^{-7}, and raw bit rate per view of 30–40 Mbps. The core network, as shown in Figure 1.2, for the case of robotic surgery, communicates with the help of 5G base stations (BSs), the communications parameters being the position or velocity, along with the force and vibration calibration values for the robotic probe. The audio and video transmissions along with haptic feedback also need to be monitored

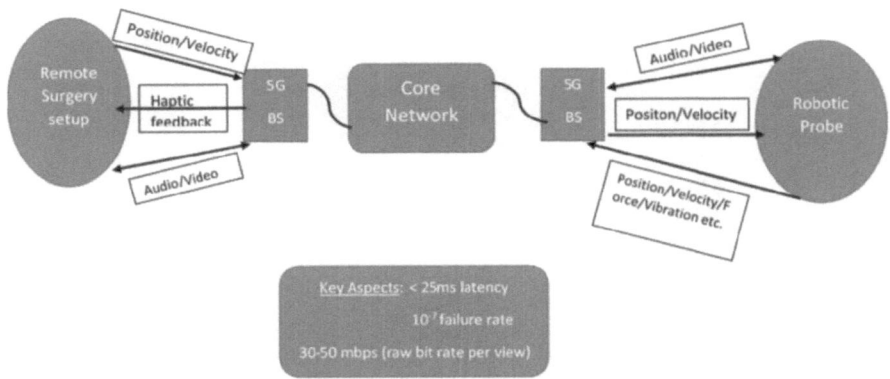

FIGURE 1.2 A generic 5G communication network based architecture depicting remote surgery healthcare application with key aspects. (Adapted from [5, 6].)

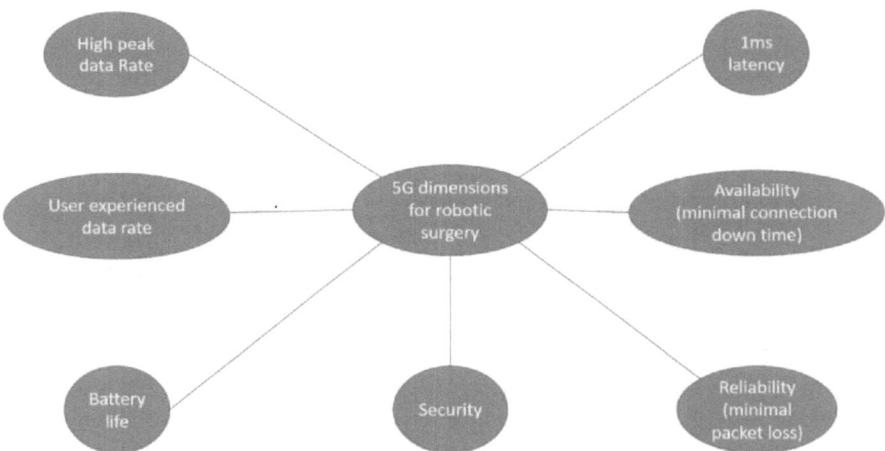

FIGURE 1.3 The dimensions for robotic surgery utilizing the 5G network architecture for applications in healthcare.

for complete communication transmission and to ensure the reliability of the communication process, in general.

Figure 1.3 gives the various dimensions of robotic surgery while utilizing the 5G network architecture. The various parameters that play an important role in deciding the network and are expected for utilizing the 5G network architecture for the robotic surgery applications are as follows.

- High peak data rate translating to a higher user–experienced data rate,
- low latency, of the order of less than 1 ms,

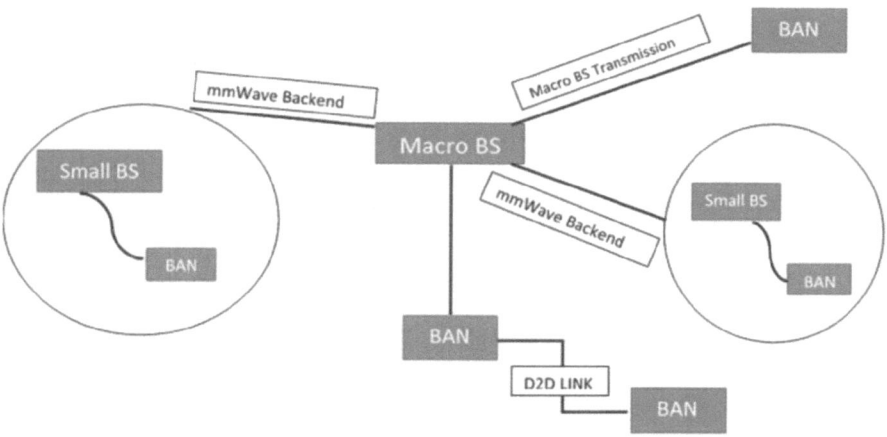

FIGURE 1.4 The 5G core network architecture for healthcare applications. (Adapted from [7, 8].)

- high reliability, namely, minimum packet loss, and high availability, which further implies, minimum connection downtime,
- higher battery life to support longer time lengths for operations, and
- highly secure network for safe transmission of patient's personal data.

Figure 1.4 depicts the suggested core network architecture of 5G for applications in healthcare. There can be various body area networks (BANs) connected to the BSs which can be small BSs serving a pico-cell or macro BSs. Further, the communication links between the BANs can be D2D [9–11] links and the communication links between the BSs can be millimeter wave based links at the back end. The 5G and beyond networks are essentially heterogeneous networks that are amalgamations of different communication networks requiring compatible communication protocols, accessibility of radio resources, interoperability of the various telecommunication operators, and compatibility between various hardware devices operating at different frequencies and power levels.

To ensure quality of service and quality of experience for the end user these challenges need to be overcome for seamless connectivity across different technologies and real user experience for critical applications in healthcare and other fields. D2D communication is one such promising technology envisaged to be an important part of the future wireless networks as it provides advantages such as offloading the traffic from the network by proposing a direct communication between the devices in proximity, bypassing the network infrastructure.

The mobile healthcare architecture is depicted in Figure 1.5, where possible interactions between various networks are described to achieve the implementation of mobile healthcare in a real and true sense. The interactions with the mobile health data are coordinated through a central platform managed on the cloud, described as the mobile health cloud platform. This mobile health cloud platform is connected to

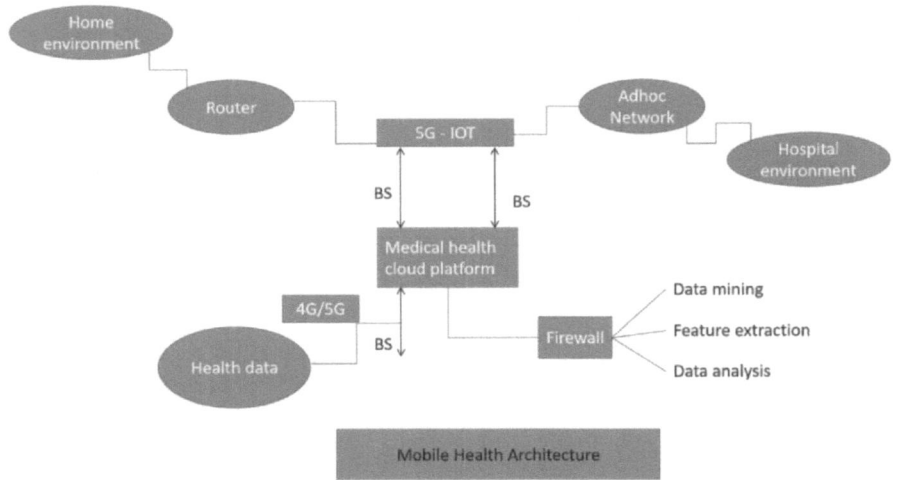

FIGURE 1.5   A generic architecture for the mobile health applications showing interactions between the 5G-IoT, cloud platform, ad hoc networks and user networks based in the home environment. (Adapted from Ref. [8].)

the health data server through the BS using 4G or 5G technology as per availability and to ensure security, the processing of data involving data mining, data analysis, and feature extraction operations is protected by firewalls as depicted in Figure 1.5. Further, the mobile healthcare cloud platform interacts with the hospital servers and the end users' home environments through 5G BS and internet-of-things (IoT) devices. The interaction with the hospital environment is through the ad hoc network and the end user can interact with the mobile healthcare platform via a router connected to the 5G–IoT device.

1.3   AI WITH 5G IN SMART HEALTHCARE

Conventional healthcare systems have been disrupted since the advent of technologies relying on the modalities of biomedical sensors, information networks, and wireless communication systems. Given the increased focus of the research community and industrial experts on reducing the capex and opex costs of healthcare for end–patients, the utilization of distributed healthcare systems has eased the lives of millions of patients for whom access to early diagnosis and treatment was a far-fetched reality [12]. Critically, a significant role in this disruption was achieved by utilizing the vantage of IoMT (Internet of Medical Things), which is not a single stream of research components or methodologies, but rather a diverse amalgamation of medical devices, sensors, and mobile applications, on which several hybrid SaaS (software as a service)-enabled business solutions rely, by means of innovative startups leading the transformation of healthcare. Briefly, the core principle that IoMT relies on is multimodal monitoring for early threat assessment leading to the steps required for early diagnosis, easier treatment, and better prevention, all the while keeping the stakeholders (patients, healthcare workers, and doctors) in a feedback connected loop.

A technical overview of IoMT would result in a generalized positive consensus on the approach given its primary reliance on interconnected devices. However, developers and experts in the field of Industry 4.0, 5G, and AI would prefer to refer to such a consensus as a layman's understanding of a rather complicated and perplexing field. Troubles emerge as we dig deep into this field, especially when taking into consideration how the reliance on interconnected devices requires a near-real-time analysis and insight generation on high-frequency long-term observational medical data collected from various data points [14]. Also, provided that the uses of IoMT are constantly on the rise, the question of ensuring a single-digit millisecond latency rate and massive bandwidth of conduction for tele surgery, and so on., becomes a question worth addressing. Although various startups, businesses, and research institutions across the globe have proposed proprietary AI-enabled 5G architectures for smart healthcare, the above questions continue to exist that require focused and intensive collaborations between industry and academia in the long run.

1.3.1 INDUSTRY APPLICATIONS: 5G ENABLED TELEMEDICINE

A real-case study of the existing impact of AI-enabled 5G solutions in smart healthcare is the rise of telemedicine. Given the lack of dexterity both theoretically and practically of AI-use cases, there continues to exist a confusion that associates the connection of AI and Big Data with personalized (also known as – precision) medicines [12]. This is far from reality, especially when one realizes the role played by the technical capacities of 5G in enabling the successful existence of precision medicines. To clearly understand the role played by 5G, it is better to contrast the state of personalized medicines backed by 4G and 4G LTE (long term evolution)–Advanced capacities, which became a common ground for limited bandwidth, slow stochastic transmission speed (around 50 Mbps even for LTE Advanced, especially when, theoretically, speeds like 300 Mbps exist). These are a summarized description of the major issues faced. There are consequences of the instability at high speed, and inefficient super-low latency interventions. Hence, it becomes clear that data transfer wasn't the only reason for the revocation of the implementation of 4G LTE for precision medicines [13].

Consequently, the obvious question is: what is the scenario for telemedicine with 5G? As concluded by various research papers and industry case studies, precision medicines have evolved to become "telemedicine", namely, massive medical devices connected to centralized cloud-computing platforms which, without network congestion, can provide an immersive and delay–free experience of healthcare in the comfort of the home [14]. Given the extensive framework of telemedicine, the addition of a 4k or 8k monitor with 360 degree virtual reality (VR) not only allows for the formulation of strategies for better treatment but also allows for the provision of immediate diagnosis, and all of this whilst utilizing the technical advantages of 5G and its ongoing revolution in terms of low-latency video delivery and streaming, extreme high-resolution medical rendering, and treatment-critical intervention [15].

1.3.2   Potential Pitfalls of 5G and its Possible Implications

Research studies and industry-based surveys have shown significant agreement in taking the view that the major pitfall of 5G is the speed of data transfer [16]. The view is often wrongly taken that the role of 5G, and other future improvements is to increase the speed of data transfer. This has resulted in misaligned expectations of this technology, whose only major selling point is to provide lower latency and higher bandwidth than 4G LTE Advanced [18]. Consequently, as these expectations go unchecked, public behavior impacts the 5G service as expectations from the service differ significantly from what the service offers. Many people concurrently access the networks hoping to utilize higher data transfer rates only to be left disappointed [17]. Though it might appear to be a hindrance, it is also considered that this excessive misaligned expectation can actually work in favor of 5G as more devices attempting to be a part of the network would require more connection nodes on a network which in turn causes the network to increase data transfer speeds in order to meet benchmarks of lower latency than 4G [19].

1.3.3   What Is Smart Healthcare?

The concept of smart healthcare came to the fore with the development of information technology. Healthcare which uses smart technologies such as big data, wearable devices, IoT, and AI, to name but a few, is described as smart healthcare in the literature. Smart technology is needed in healthcare to make it efficient, convenient, and personalized. With the advancement of information and technology, conventional medicine and the healthcare sector also gradually began to digitize and introduce the concepts of preventive healthcare rather than only focusing on disease treatment. Various features of 5G such as fast data transmission with low latency, large bandwidth, intelligently make use of physical resources and intelligence at the edges of the network making 5G more popular for smart healthcare.

1.4   APPLICATIONS OF 5G IN HEALTHCARE AND OPEN CHALLENGES

Although 5G has various features starting with huge bandwidth to support critical and high demand services, such as augmented and virtual reality, an important issue is connectivity, since the continuously growing number of devices generates congestion in the communication channels. IoT devices are extremely heterogeneous in their computing capabilities, communication protocols and application fields and due to this wide diversity and extremely varying capabilities it is difficult to collaborate and to access all information necessary for ensuring their optimal efficiency. Figure 1.6 shows some of the opportunities and open challenges in 5G healthcare applications. Major challenges are the high cost, different coverage in urban and rural areas, and cyber security based issues.

The various opportunities available with 5G lie in support to upload and download large files, its use as a means to perform robotic surgery, and personalized patient services, and so forth.

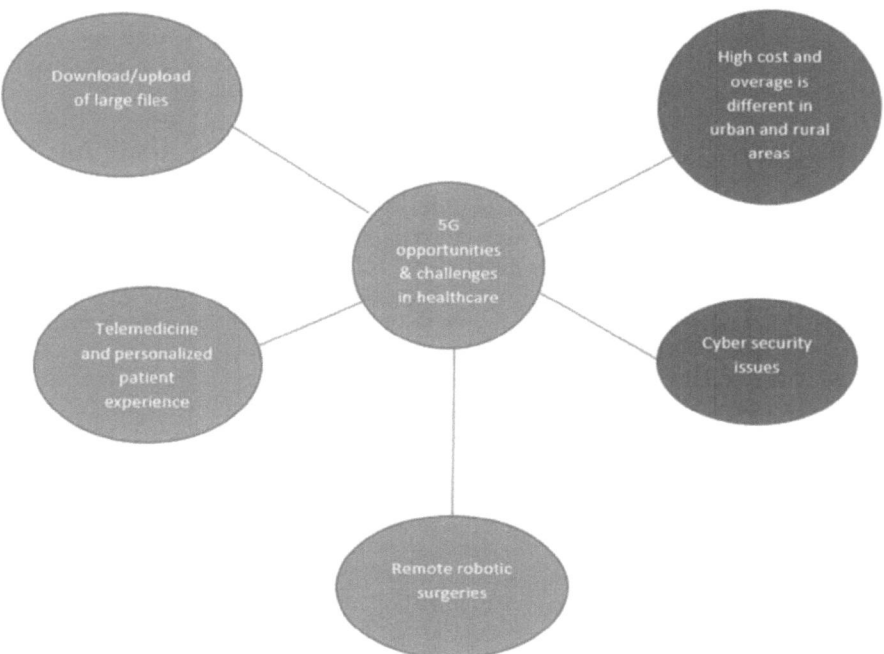

FIGURE 1.6 5G Opportunities and open challenges in healthcare applications. (Adapted from Ref. [20].)

1.5 CONCLUSION

Recent advances in the field of Artificial intelligence and 5G communication, has created new possibilities for the healthcare domain. 5G technology has begun to show great advantages in improving intelligent hospital services, allowing automatic patient monitoring, performing precise remote surgical operations, promoting the rational allocation of quality medical resources, and efficient management of wearable devices and monitoring devices carried by patients. In this chapter, a brief overview has been provided of the 5G network and its specific application to healthcare, and its advantages and disadvantages. Further, the concept of smart healthcare and the focus towards artificial intelligence providing solutions to many computational challenges and efficient resource allocation has been given. In our view, 5G technology will revolutionize the way we use healthcare services and will lead to better and fair allocation of healthcare services in society.

REFERENCES

1. 5G in healthcare, PWC report. Online. www.pwc.com/gx/en/industries/tmt/5g/pwc-5g-in-healthcare.pdf
2. Stracuzzi, M. "Revolutionary Use Cases of 5G in Healthcare", 2020. Online. www.telit.com/blog/4-revolutionary-use-cases-5g-healthcare/

3. Understanding the opportunities for operators in healthcare, Ericsson report. Online. www.ericsson.com/en/networks/trending/insights-and-reports/5g-healthcare
4. Liu, E., Effiok, E. and Hitchcock, J. "Survey on health care applications in 5G networks," *IET Communications*, vol. 14, no. 7, pp. 1073–1080, 2020.
5. Ahad, A., Tahir, M., and Yau, K. A. "5G-based smart healthcare network: Architecture, taxonomy, challenges and future research directions," *IEEE Access*, vol. 7, pp. 100747–100762, 2019.
6. Soldani, D. et al., "5G Mobile Systems for Healthcare," *IEEE 85th Vehicular Technology Conference (VTC Spring)*, Sydney, NSW, pp. 1–5, 2017.
7. Rao, K. "The Path to 5G for Health Care," *IEEE Future Networks*. Online. https://fut urenetworks.ieee.org/images/files/pdf/applications/5G--Health-Care030518.pdf
8. Thuemmler, C. et al., "A new generation of e-health systems powered by 5G," White paper in Wireless World Research Forum, Nov. 2016.
9. Joshi, S., and Mallik, R. K. "Coverage probability analysis in a device-to-device network: Interference functional and Laplace transform based approach," *IEEE Communications Letters*, vol. 23, no. 3, pp. 466–469, Mar. 2019.
10. Joshi, S., and Mallik, R. K. "Coverage and interference in D2D networks with Poisson cluster process," *IEEE Communications Letters*, vol. 22, no. 5, pp. 1098–1101, May 2018.
11. Joshi, S., and Mallik, R. K. "Analysis of dedicated and shared device-to-device communication in cellular networks over Nakagami-m fading channels," *IET Communications*, vol. 11, no. 10, pp. 1600–1609, Jul. 2017.
12. Li, D. "5G and intelligence medicine—how the next generation of wireless technology will reconstruct healthcare?" *Precision Clinical Medicine*, vol. 2, no. 4, pp. 205–208, 2019.
13. Song, Y., Jiang, J., Wang, X., Yang, D. and Bai, C. "Prospect and application of Internet of Things technology for prevention of SARIs." *Clinical eHealth*, vol. 3, pp. 1–4, 2020.
14. Li, X., Guo, L., Sun, L., Yue, P. W. and Xu, H. "Tele ultrasound for the COVID-19 pandemic: A statement from China." *Advanced Ultrasound In Diagnosis and Therapy*, vol. 4, no.2, pp. 50–56, 2020.
15. Rathore, H. and Kumar, A. "Reduction of peak average power ratio for FBMC waveform with P-PTS technique." *International Journal of Sensors Wireless Communications and Control*, vol. 10, no. 1, pp. 47–54, 2020.
16. Zakrzewska, A., Ruepp, S. and Berger, M. S. "Towards converged 5G mobile networks-challenges and current trends". In *Proceedings of the 2014 ITU kaleidoscope academic conference: Living in a converged world-Impossible without standards?* (pp. 39–45). IEEE, June 2014.
17. Boccardi, F., Heath, R. W., Lozano, A., Marzetta, T. L. and Popovski, P. "Five disruptive technology directions for 5G." *IEEE Communications Magazine*, vol. 52, no. 2, pp. 74–80, 2014.
18. Agyapong, P. K., Iwamura, M., Staehle, D., Kiess, W. and Benjebbour, A. "Design considerations for a 5G network architecture." *IEEE Communications Magazine*, vol. 52, no. 11, pp. 65–75, 2014.
19. West, D. M. "How 5G technology enables the health internet of things." Brookings Center for Technology Innovation, 3, 1–20, 2016. Online. www.brookings.edu/resea rch/how-5g-technology-enables-the-health-internet-of-things/
20. Siriwardhana, Y, et al. "The role of 5G for digital healthcare against COVID-19 pandemic: Opportunities and challenges." *ICT Express*, 2020.

2 Advances of 5G Wireless Communication Systems in Healthcare Informatics

Ajay Yadav, Rashmi, Rahul Mukherjee,
Ashok Kumar, Jitendra Kumar Deegwal,
Ghanshyam Singh, and Harpreet Vohra

CONTENTS

2.1   INTRODUCTION

Internet of Things (IoT) applications in the healthcare sector have tremendous opportunities. During pandemic times, physical contact needs to be avoided and maintaining social distance is essential. IoT based healthcare systems can be considered for the control of pandemics similar to Covid-19, in the future. For the extensive use of IoT focused healthcare, 5G wireless communication systems are used all over the world. In many advanced countries such as China, USA, and South Korea, 5G is already deployed in some cities, and it is in the implementation stage in countries such as India. An IoT based system using artificial intelligence (AI) can control a pandemic to a large extent. It can help to prevent the spread of Covid-19 in the following ways [1, 2]:

- Secure public safety systems using computer vision technology,
- Drone usage for delivery of items and sanitization,
- Tracing people with smartphone-based apps using GPS location,
- Limiting use of public transport using artificial intelligence empowered platforms.

With the IoT, patients who are suffering from diseases such Parkinson's, and Alzheimer's can be monitored from remote areas [3]. It aids patients who are alone and who need immediate help [4]. IoT based healthcare solutions manage hospital equipment, patients in a timely fashion, and help to avoid emergency situations [5]. For example, glucose levels can be monitored continuously for a diabetic patient using the IoT from a remote location [6]. Vedaei et al. [1], explain that researchers have developed an IoT framework for the measurement of body temperature, blood oxygen saturation level, heart rate, and for the observation of coughing patterns of patients. Moreover, patients can be tracked by GPS location devices. Further, the collected data can be uploaded to the cloud, and data analysis and decision making can be performed by machine learning algorithms both as supervised and unsupervised learning algorithms.

In Figure 2.1, the 5G communication system architecture is shown, where data from the various sensors is collected, and passed through the local processing unit (LPU) to the body sensor network (BSN) server via an access point [7, 8]. The various sensors are installed for determining electroencephalogram (EEG), electrocardiogram (ECG), and electromyogram (EMG) signals and for the measurement of blood pressure (BP), temperature and motion of the patient. The collected data from the sensors is transmitted to a smart phone or microcontroller, which acts as a local processing unit (LPU). The processed data is further sent to a BSN cloud server via an access point such as a Wi-Fi router or base transceiver station (BTS). In a BSN server, stored data can be analysed using machine learning algorithms such as linear discriminant analysis (LDA) and principal component analysis (PCA) [9] or real-time data can also be live streamed on the Thing Speak Cloud or through a smartphone app such as Blynk. The following steps are used in LDA:

Step1: The scaled data point is defined as:
Variable_N = (existing variable-average of all variables)/ (standard deviation of all variables).
Step 2: Generate a covariance matrix.
Step 3: Find eigenvalues and eigenvectors.
Step 4: Calculate the principal components.

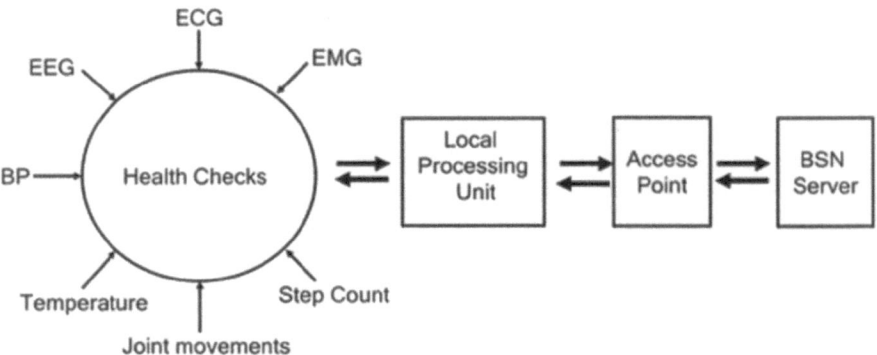

FIGURE 2.1 IoT-based 5G communication architecture for body sensor network.

This algorithm generates small data from the large data set without loss of important features.

For a secure healthcare system, a secure social IoT health framework with a physical layer cryptography scheme is proposed [10]. The proposed scheme is for BSN applications. In [11], medical certificates are issued by the IoT based healthcare system using blockchain technology. Blockchain is also used for payment verification processes in the e-healthcare system [12, 13]. A blockchain based 5G architecture is proposed in [14]. Several researchers have proposed blockchain, cloud computing, and software defined network (SDN) usage in the healthcare sector for secure, low latency, low cost, and reliable communication systems [15–19].

2.2   HEALTHCARE-INTERNET OF THINGS (H-IOT)

The H-IoT term is coined for medical science applications. In the H-IoT system, the various health resources are connected over the internet for exchange of data. In the healthcare sector, a huge amount of data is accumulated from the various sensors. Machine learning approaches can be used with these data sets for intelligent decision making by doctors in hospitals. The layered architecture of H-IoT is given in Table 2.1.

The H-IoT layers are implemented using technologies as shown in Figure 2.2. Every node is associated with sensor module for data collection. The various nodes in the network can be identified with a unique ID (UID). So, identification of the node is feasible with RFID technology. The IoT nodes communicate with each other using various communication technologies such as Bluetooth, Zigbee, Wi-Fi, 4G/5G, and the like. The communication technology depends on various parameters such as data rate, distance between nodes, communication system budget, power usage, and so forth. For locating the nodes in the network, a global positioning system (GPS) can be used which detects the sensor node location. The collected data is uploaded on the cloud server. The analytical results from the cloud server can be evaluated by the doctor using a smartphone app or web browser.

M. Haghi et al. proposed a healthcare-based platform for monitoring physiological and environment parameters [20]. Further, a wearable sensor patch which consumes less power and light in weight is developed in [21] for the measurement of ECG, photoplethysmography (PPG), and body temperature. An efficient transceiver is demonstrated [22] using orthogonal frequency division multiplexing (OFDM) technology and data compression.

TABLE 2.1
H-IoT Layered Architecture

Data Collection Layer	Collection of data from the various sensors on the patient's body
Data Storage Layer	Storage of large amount of data
Data Processing Layer	Various computing algorithms are implemented on the cloud

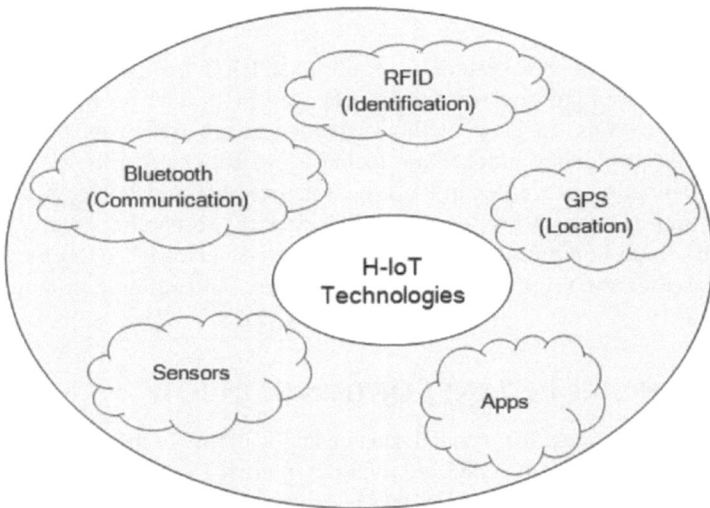

FIGURE 2.2   Technologies used in different layers of H-IoT.

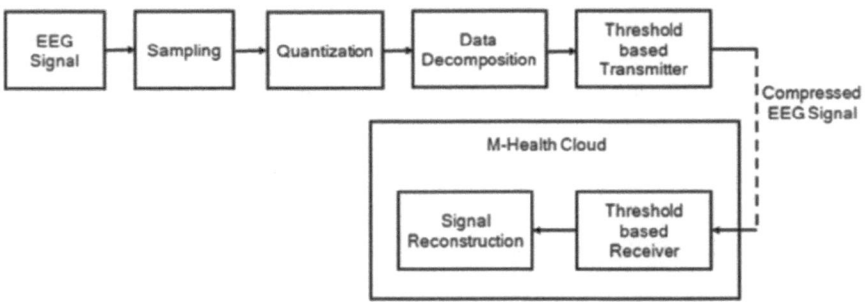

FIGURE 2.3   System model.

Figure 2.3 shows the translation of an EEG signal to an M-health cloud end-to-end system. The EEG signal is obtained through an EEG headset attached to a patient's head. The signal is sampled, quantized, and decomposed for the application of the compression scheme. The compressed signal is transmitted and received by the proposed threshold-based transmitter and receiver, respectively. With this efficient design of transceiver, the communication system achieves excellent performance with reference to data reduction gain, reduced system complexity, and signal distortion. The data is compressed by up to 50%, with 0% distortion and sample error rate [22].

Researchers have proposed various technological tools for healthcare diagnostic tools and sensors [23]. The advances in materials and processes have also been explained which led to precision in diagnostic data, and reduction in the price and size of healthcare products.

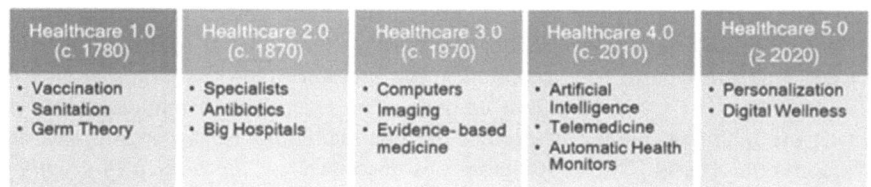

FIGURE 2.4   Healthcare transformation.

2.3   HEALTHCARE TECHNOLOGY TRANSFORMATION

The history of the healthcare system is related to the history of medicine as depicted in Figure 2.4. In medicine 1.0, doctors prescribed medicines and these medicines were natural herbs. Healthcare 1.0 involved solving major health problems using intelligent public health decisions such vaccination and sanitization. With the discovery of antibiotics and X-ray machines, the concept of specialization in diagnostics techniques and of big hospitals started in healthcare. This is referred to as healthcare 2.0. In healthcare 2.0, mass production of medicines and surgical instruments by industry took place. This was followed by evidence-based medicine in healthcare 3.0 where surgical robots, navigation surgery, and image recognition are the main features. With advancements in communication and microelectronics technology, advanced medical diagnosis, and treatments such as chemotherapy, telematic therapy, and intelligent implants for the body are an important part of healthcare 4.0. Wearables such as smart watches consist of multiple sensors for collecting data. The patient is monitored and diagnosed by a doctor from the physiological data. This data is further analysed using artificial intelligence (AI) and machine learning. An IoT device with AI faces the following challenges at the communication layer level [24]:

- Data transmission without loss,
- Less congestion in transmission channels,
- Cost-effectiveness,
- Data retrieval from the packets lost in the internet traffic,
- Machine to machine (M2M) communication.

These challenges are addressed in the 5G communication system. With 5G communication, the personalized healthcare model, where individual well-being is the priority plays an important role in medicine 5.0 or healthcare 5.0.

2.4   SECURE H-IOT

The data collected from wearable medical implants and smart watches can be monitored by a doctor in real-time and uploaded onto a cloud server for further analysis. The collected data is spatial and temporal. The spatial data is used by pharmaceutical industries for the research and development of drugs and medical devices. Doctors monitor and diagnose individual patients from the temporal data. The patient data can be retrieved by an eavesdropper in the communication channel or from device storage. So, security of patient data is very essential in H-IoT. Several cryptographic algorithms have been reported in the literature [24–27]. Cryptography is a current encryption technology that comprises of several mathematical operations. It was originally developed to protect the confidentiality of diplomatic and military communications [28]. Cryptography is described as *"the branch of cryptology concerned with the development of encryption and decryption methods to ensure the security and authentication of data"*. Encryption and decryption are the most basic functions of cryptography [28]. Encryption refers to a conversion process whereby plain text is processed and converted into secured and coded text so that it is difficult for an unauthorised party to recover the actual message whereas decryption is a process whereby ciphertext (coded text) is turned into the original text. Both features are used to protect messages from being viewed by people who aren't authorised to see them [29, 30].

Blockchain technology is used for crypto-security, and for transparent and secure data networks [7]. With healthcare 4.0 and blockchain 3.0 data network processes, a smart healthcare system has been designed and implemented. The various healthcare 4.0 processes are IoT, industrial IoT, cloud, cognitive, artificial intelligence, quantum computing, fog, and edge computing, and the like. Optimized algorithms are implemented on healthcare 4.0 technologies along with the secure blockchain decentralized data network.

Ahmad F. Subahi [31] proposed the architecture, design, and recommendation for an edge based IoT healthcare management system. There is redistribution of workload between two subsystems: 1) A sub-system for the monitoring of assignments, and 2) A sub-system for the record keeping of medical data. These subsystems interact with SQL and non-SQL database management systems [31]. In [32], "All4Health" IoT architecture is described which is superior to existing architecture in terms of scalability, fault tolerance, dependableness, adaptability, and interoperability. Further, a novel scheduling scheme for data streaming in edge-devices is demonstrated where a task level re-timing methodology called R-CTG (Conditional Task Graph) is used with non-linear programming dependent scheduling [33]. In H-IoT security, the various challenges are [34]:

- Maintaining the standardization,
- Internet interaction,
- Scalability in networks,
- Data management,
- Controlling security protocols,
- Embedded systems,
- Integration of health data.

2.5   H-IOT COMMUNICATION PROTOCOLS

Communication protocols are used for the transfer of data between heterogeneous devices in H-IoT. The various standards and protocols are formed by the World Wide Web Consortium (W3C), the Institute of Electrical and Electronics Engineers

(IEEE), the European Telecommunications Standards Institute (ETSI), the Internet Engineering Task Force (IETF), and Electronic Product Code (EPC) global. The communication protocols can be categorized into three types [34]:

1. **Application protocols:** where, constrained application protocol (CoAP), the data distribution service, message queue telemetry transport (MQTT), extensible messaging and presence protocol (XMPP), and advanced message queuing protocol are the various protocols used in H-IoT based 5G communication system.
2. **Service discovery protocols:** DNS service discovery (DNS-SD), and multicast domain name system (mDNS) are the protocols used in resource rich H-IoT.
3. **Infrastructure protocols:** are as follows:
    1. Routing protocol for low power and lossy networks,
    2. Low-rate wireless personal area network (LR-WPAN),
    3. Low power wireless personal area network (6LoWPAN),
    4. Bluetooth low energy (BLE),
    5. EPCglobal,
    6. Long Term Evolution-Advanced (LTE-A),
    7. Z-wave.

2.6 CONCLUSION

The healthcare sector is a very important aspect of the 5G communication system. H-IoT will play a very important function in shaping the future of patients in healthcare 5.0. A 5G communication system with BSN will lead to personalized well-being in future. The various communication layers and the corresponding technologies make us understand the H-IoT. H-IoT faces various security challenges. The solutions of these security issues are proposed by various researchers. Numerous communication protocols are proposed in application, service, and infrastructure of H-IoT. The use of H-IoT devices and diagnostic tools will increase in the future very rapidly. H-IoT is an integral part of the 5G communication network.

REFERENCES

1. Vedaei, S. S., Fotovvat, A., Mohebbian, M. R. *et al.* "COVID-SAFE: An IoT-based system for automated health monitoring and surveillance in post-pandemic life." *IEEE Access*, 8, 188538–51, 2020.
2. Pasluosta, C. F., Gassner, H., Winkler, J., Klucken, J., Eskofier, B. M. "An emerging era in the management of Parkinson's disease: wearable technologies and the internet of things." *IEEE Journal of Biomedical and Health Informatics*, 19, no. 6: 1873–81, 2015.
3. Laplante, P. A., and Laplante R. "The internet of things in healthcare: potential applications and challenges." *IT Professional*, 18, no. 3: 2–4, 2016.
4. Pandey, P. and Litoriya, R. "Elderly care through unusual behaviour detection: A disaster management approach using IoT and Intelligence." *IBM Journal of Research and Development*, 64, nos. 1–2: 1–11, 2019.

5. Kang, S., Baek, H., Jung, E., Hwang, H., and Yoo S. "Survey on the demand for adoption of Internet of Things (IoT)-based services in hospitals: Investigations of nurses' perceptions in a tertiary university hospital." *Applied Nursing Research*, 47: 18–23, 2019.

6. Chang, S-H., Chiang, R-D., Wu, S-J., and Chang, W-T. "A context-aware, interactive M-health system for diabetics." *IT Professional*, 18, no. 3: 14–22, 2016.

7. Kumar, A., Krishnamurthi, R., Nayyar, A., Sharma, K., Grover, V., and Hossain, E. "A novel smart healthcare design, simulation, and implementation using healthcare 4.0 processes." *IEEE Access*, 8: 118433–71, 2020.

8. Gope, P., Gheraibia, Y., Kabir, S., and Sikdar, B. "A secure IoT-based modern healthcare system with fault-tolerant decision making process." *IEEE Journal of Biomedical and Health Informatics*, 25, no. 3: 862–73, 2021.

9. Bhardwaj, H. K., Agarwal, A., and Chamola, V. *et al.* "A review on the role of machine learning in enabling IoT based healthcare applications." *IEEE Access*, 9: 38859–90, 2021.

10. Hao, P. and Wang, X. "A PHY-aided secure IoT healthcare system with collaboration of social networks." *2017 IEEE 86th Vehicular Technology Conference (VTC-Fall)*: 1–6, 2017.

11. Namasudra, S., Sharma, P., Crespo, R. G., and Shanmuganathan, V. "Blockchain-based medical certificate generation and verification for IoT-based healthcare systems." *IEEE Consumer Electronics Magazine*: 1–1, 2022.

12. Ray, P. P., Dash, D., Salah, K., and Kumar, N. "Blockchain for IoT-based healthcare: Background, consensus, platforms, and use cases." *IEEE Systems Journal*, 15, no. 1: 85–94, 2021.

13. Ray, P. P., Kumar, N., and Dash, D. "BLWN: Blockchain-based lightweight simplified payment verification in IoT-assisted e-Healthcare." *IEEE Systems Journal*, 15, no. 1: 134–45, 2021.

14. Khujamatov, K., Reypnazarov, E., Akhmedov, N., and Khasanov, D. "Blockchain for 5G healthcare architecture." *2020 International Conference on Information Science and Communications Technologies (ICISCT)*: 1–5, 2021.

15. Ren, J., Li, J., Liu, H., and Qin, T. "Task offloading strategy with emergency handling and blockchain security in SDN-empowered and fog-assisted healthcare IoT." *Tsinghua Science and Technology*, 27, no. 4: 760–76, 2022.

16. Yogeshwar, A. and Kamalakkannan, S. "Building dynamic permutation based privacy preservation model with block chain technology for IoT healthcare sector." *2022 International Conference on Advanced Computing Technologies and Applications (ICACTA)*: 1–8, 2022.

17. Gunanidhi, G. S. and Krishnaveni, R. "Improved security blockchain for IoT based healthcare monitoring system." *2022 Second International Conference on Artificial Intelligence and Smart Energy (ICAIS)*: 1244–47, 2022.

18. Kumar, R., Kumar, P., Tripathi, R., Gupta, G. P., Najumal Islam, A. K. M., and Shorfuzzaman, M. "Permissioned blockchain and deep-learning for secure and efficient data sharing in industrial healthcare systems." *IEEE Transactions on Industrial Informatics,* 2022.

19. Liu, Y., Shan, G., Liu, Y., Alghamdi, A., Alam, I., and Biswas, S. "Blockchain bridges critical national infrastructures: E-healthcare data migration perspective." *IEEE Access*, 10: 28509–19, 2022.

20. Haghi, M., Neubert, S., and Geissler, A. *et al.* "A flexible and pervasive IoT-based healthcare platform for physiological and environmental parameters monitoring." *IEEE Internet of Things Journal*, 7, no. 6: 5628–47, 2020.

21. Wu, T., Wu, F., Qiu, C., Redouté, J-M., and Yuce, M. R. "A rigid-flex wearable health monitoring sensor patch for IoT-connected healthcare applications." *IEEE Internet of Things Journal*, 7, no. 8: 6932–45, 2020.
22. Abdellatif, A. A., Khafagy, M. G., Mohamed, A., and Chiasserini, C. "EEG-based transceiver design with data decomposition for healthcare IoT applications." *IEEE Internet of Things Journal*, 5, no. 5: 3569–79, 2018.
23. Knickerbocker, J. U., Budd, R., Dang, B. *et al.* "Heterogeneous integration technology demonstrations for future healthcare, IoT, and AI computing solutions." *2018 IEEE 68th Electronic Components and Technology Conference (ECTC)*: 1519–28, 2018.
24. Rezaeibagha, F., Mu, Y., Huang, K., and Chen, L. "Secure and efficient data aggregation for IoT monitoring systems." *IEEE Internet of Things Journal*, 8, no. 10: 8056–63, 2021.
25. Rezaeibagha, F., Mu, Y., Huang, X., Yang, W., and Huang, K. "Fully secure lightweight certificateless signature scheme for IIoT." *IEEE Access*, 7: 144433–43, 2019.
26. Hong, J., Liu, B., Sun, Q. et al. "A combined public-key scheme in the case of attribute-based for wireless body area networks." *Wireless Networks*, 25: 845–59, 2019.
27. Tang, W., Ren, J., Deng, K., and Zhang, Y. "Secure data aggregation of lightweight E-healthcare IoT devices with fair incentives." *IEEE Internet of Things Journal*, 6, no. 5: 8714–26, 2019.
28. Meyer, C. H. "Cryptography-a state of the art review." *Proceedings. VLSI and Computer Peripherals. COMPEURO 89*: 4/150-4/154, 1989.
29. Massey, J. L. "An introduction to contemporary cryptology." *Proceedings of the IEEE*, 76, no. 5: 533–49, 1988.
30. Data Encryption Standard, Federal Information Processing Standard (FIPS) Publication 46, National Bureau of Standards, U.S. Department of Commerce, Washington, DC (January 1977).
31. Subahi, A. F. "Edge-based IoT medical record system: Requirements, recommendations and conceptual design." *IEEE Access*, 7: 94150–59, 2019.
32. Plageras, A. P., Psannis, K. E., Ishibashi, Y., and Kim, B-G. "IoT-based surveillance system for ubiquitous healthcare." *IECON 2016-42nd Annual Conference of the IEEE Industrial Electronics Society*: 6226–30, 2016.
33. Tariq, U. U., Ali, H., Liu, L., Hardy, J., Kazim, M., and Ahmed W. "Energy-aware scheduling of streaming applications on edge-devices in IoT-based healthcare." *IEEE Transactions on Green Communications and Networking*, 5, no. 2: 803–15, 2021.
34. Bhuiyan, M. N., Rahman, M. M., Billah, M. M., and Saha, D. "Internet of Things (IoT): A review of its enabling technologies in healthcare applications, standards protocols, security, and market opportunities." *IEEE Internet of Things Journal*, 8, no. 13: 10474–98, 2021.

3 Beamforming in Massive MIMO Communications for 5G Technology

Ahmad Kamal Hassan, Muhammad Moinuddin, Abdulrahman U. Alsaggaf, and Ubaid M. Al-Saggaf

CONTENTS

3.1 INTRODUCTION

Massive multiple-input multiple-out (mMIMO) constitutes a base station (BS) having a much higher number of antenna elements compared to the total number of users in its vicinity [1]. mMIMO systems are efficient in spectral and power fronts, where the infrastructure change is required mainly at the BS instead of mobile stations (MS) [1], [2]. Hence, a mMIMO system renders a better network capable of delivering the performance objectives of the emerging generation of communication systems [3], [4].

In the design of mMIMO systems, a consideration of partial channel state information (CSI) is often considered following the exact closed-form expression of key performance indicators (KPIs) under maximum ratio transmission (MRT), or zero forcing (ZF) transmit beamforming schemes [5–7], or by considering perfect CSI accessibility [8]. Also, several approximate results for KPIs are given in [9] by employing asymptotic schemes using order statistics and extreme-value theory referred in [10]. Furthermore, in the downlink system and along these lines, the impact of transmission antenna spatial correlation on sum rate capacity is postulated in [11]. A closed-form expression of capacity of the multipath independent Rayleigh fading channel is given in [12]. A model without consideration of co-channel interference is analyzed in [13] using the characteristic function of MIMO with the assumption of no instantaneous CSI at the transmission side.

DOI: 10.1201/9781003368311-3

Motivated by the discussion above, in this chapter we provide a more comprehensive framework for analysis and design of beamforming weights based on the recently introduced approach of indefinite quadratic forms [14]. The content of this chapter in mainly based on these works given in [14–18]. More specifically, we provide a framework for the canonical formulation of signal-to-interference-plus-noise ratio (SINR) for an mMIMO system, characterization of outage probability (OP) using only statistical CSI availability at the transmission side, and a design of transmit beamforming weights used in the minimization of the derived expression OP under power loading constraints.

The organization after the introduction is as follows. In Section 3.2, we outline a system model of mMIMO, and, in Section 3.3, we characterize the OP of an mMIMO system. In Section 3.4, we derive a transmit beamforming design using a constrained optimization objective whose solution is obtained using an iterative method. In Section 3.5, we authenticate our results using simulation. Finally, in Section 3.6, we summarize our work.

3.2 SYSTEM MODEL

We consider a downlink mMIMO scenario adopted from [16] as depicted in Figure 3.1, where BS having N transmit antennas communicate to K user devices having a single antenna element. Herein, $N > K$ is considered as per the mMIMO scheme. Among the total number of users identified as K, we select the kth user. Next, s_k is the data symbol which is multiplied with a transmit beam-vector w_k of dimensions $N \times 1$ at the transmission stage. We assume that s_k is normalized, that is, $E\left|s_i\right|^2 = 1$, for $\forall i$.

Now, from the aforementioned considerations, we mathematically express the signal received at the kth user as

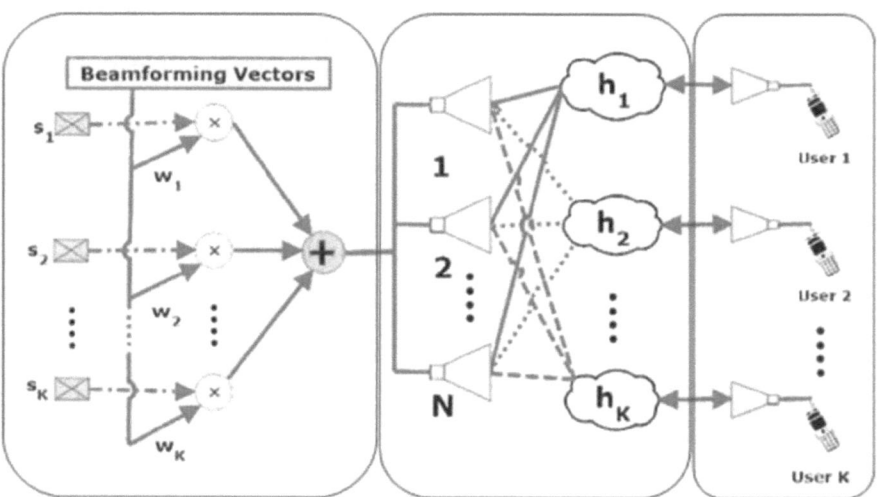

FIGURE 3.1   Block diagram of downlink multi-user mMIMO system [16].

$$y_k = \mathbf{h}_k^{\mathrm{H}} \mathbf{w}_k s_k + \sum_{i=1, i \neq k}^{K} \mathbf{h}_k^{H} \mathbf{w}_i s_i + v_k \tag{3.1}$$

where $\mathbf{h}_k^{\mathrm{H}}$ having dimension of $1 \times N$ is basically a kth channel vector, and it is a zero-mean complex and circular Gaussian channel having covariance $\mathbf{R}_k$, that is, $\mathbf{h}_k \sim CN(0, \mathbf{R}_k)$.

In Equation 3.1, the 1st term indicates the desired signal of user k, while the 2nd term is representative of the co-channel interference received, and the 3rd term is additive noise which is considered as zero-mean white noise with variance σ_k^2.

To proceed further we adopt the framework in [16] in this section. Thus, we express the instantaneous SINR as γ_k, where the subscript identifies the kth user, as follows

$$\gamma_k = \frac{\left| \boldsymbol{h}_k^H w_k \right|^2}{\sigma_k^2 + \sum_{i=1, i \neq k}^{K} \left| \boldsymbol{h}_k^H w_i \right|^2} \tag{3.2}$$

To simplify, we express γ_k as the ratio of indefinite quadratic form which yields

$$\gamma_k = \frac{\| \boldsymbol{h}_k \|^2_{w_k w_k^H}}{\sigma_k^2 + \| \boldsymbol{h}_k \|^2_{\sum_{i=1, i \neq k}^{K} w_i w_i^H}} \tag{3.3}$$

Next, we consider a whitened version of the channel, that is, $\overline{\boldsymbol{h}}_k = \boldsymbol{R}_k^{-\frac{H}{2}} \boldsymbol{h}_k$. Consequently, γ_k simplifies to

$$\gamma_k = \frac{\| \overline{\boldsymbol{h}}_k \|^2_{\boldsymbol{R}_k^{\frac{1}{2}} w_k w_k^H \boldsymbol{R}_k^{\frac{H}{2}}}}{\sigma_k^2 + \| \overline{\boldsymbol{h}}_k \|^2_{\boldsymbol{R}_k^{\frac{1}{2}} \left(\sum_{i=1, i \neq k}^{K} w_i w_i^H \right) \boldsymbol{R}_k^{\frac{H}{2}}}} \tag{3.4}$$

Note that the length of the channels is dependent on the number of antennas at the transmit side.

3.3   CHARACTERIZATION OF OUTAGE PROBABILITY

In this section, we employ IQF methodology to characterize the OP of the kth user in the K user scenario. Again, the content of this section is adopted from [16] where we employ the IQF approach, and hence characterize the OP of the kth user in the downlink Gaussian broadcast scenario. Now, using Equation 3.5 and for a given threshold γ_{th}, the CDF, that is, $\Pr(\gamma_k < \gamma)$ is expressed, for notational shortness, as $P_{k,out}(\gamma)$ and is given by:

$$P_{k,out}(\gamma) = \Pr\left(\frac{\|\bar{h}_k\|^2_{\frac{1}{R_k^2} w_k w_k^H R_k^{\frac{H}{2}}}}{\sigma_k^2 + \|\bar{h}_k\|^2_{\frac{1}{R_k^2}\left(\sum_{i=1,i\neq k}^{K} w_i w_i^H\right) R_k^{\frac{H}{2}}}} < \gamma \right) \qquad (3.5)$$

Hence, using the residue theory approach, the closed-form solution of OP for the kth user in the mMIMO downlink environment is given by

$$P_{k,out}(\gamma) = 1 - \sum_{n=1}^{N} \frac{-\lambda_n^N}{\prod_{i=1,i\neq n}^{N}(\lambda_n - \lambda_i)} \frac{1}{|\lambda_n|} e^{-\frac{\sigma_k^2 \gamma}{\lambda_n}} u\left(\frac{\sigma_k^2 \gamma}{\lambda_n} \right) \qquad (3.6)$$

where λ_n denotes the nth eigenvalue of $R_k^{\frac{1}{2}} w_k w_k^H R_k^{\frac{H}{2}} - \gamma\left(R_k^{\frac{1}{2}}\left(\sum_{i=1,i\neq k}^{K} w_i w_i^H \right) R_k^{\frac{H}{2}} \right)$,

given that all eigenvalues are distinct. On the otherhand, if the eigenvalues are repeated, then

$$P_{k,out}(\gamma_{th}) = u\left(\sigma_k^2 \gamma_{th}\right) + \sum_{l=1}^{L}\sum_{s=1}^{S} \frac{\alpha_{s,l}}{(\Gamma(s))^s} \frac{1}{|\lambda_l|^s} e^{-\frac{\sigma_k^2 \gamma_{th}}{\lambda_l}} u\left(\frac{\sigma_k^2 \gamma_{th}}{\lambda_l} \right) \qquad (3.7)$$

where $\alpha_{s,l}$ denotes the partial fraction expansion coefficients of $R_k^{\frac{1}{2}} w_k w_k^H R_k^{\frac{H}{2}} - \gamma\left(R_k^{\frac{1}{2}}\left(\sum_{i=1,i\neq k}^{K} w_i w_i^H \right) R_k^{\frac{H}{2}} \right)$, which can be evaluated using the following approach:

$$\alpha_{s,l} = \frac{1}{(S-s)!} \lim_{(j\omega+\beta)\to\frac{-1}{\lambda_l}} \frac{d^{S-s}}{d(j\omega+\beta)^{S-s}}$$

$$\times \left(\frac{1}{(j\omega+\beta)} \times \prod_{\bar{l}=1,\bar{l}\neq l}^{L} \frac{\lambda_{\bar{l}}^{\bar{S}}}{\left((j\omega+\beta)+\frac{1}{\lambda_{\bar{l}}}\right)^{\bar{S}}} \right) \qquad (3.8)$$

3.4 OPTIMIZATION OF BEAMFORMING WEIGHTS

The outage probability derived in Equation 3.6 is a non-convex function which is difficult to optimize. Thus, it is converted into a convex problem using linear scalarization (L–S). Such formulation results in Pareto optimal solutions for each of the single objective functions. This is achieved by defining a single objective function J which is formed by the linear scalar sum of the outage probabilities of all users, that is,

$$J\left(w,\gamma_{th}\right) = \sum_{k=1}^{K} c_k P_{k,out}\left(\gamma_{th}\right) \qquad (3.9)$$

where the objective function shows that it is a function of beamforming weights. To obtain an optimized solution, we propose to minimize the following constrained objective function

$$\min_{w} J\left(w,\gamma_{th}\right) = \sum_{k=1}^{K} c_k P_{k,out}\left(\gamma_{th}\right) \qquad (3.10)$$

subject to $\| w_k^2 \| = 1$

Thus, the proposed beamforming method tries to find an optimal solution by minimizing a linearized sum of all users' outage probabilities while constraining their beamforming powers to unity.

3.5   SIMULATION RESULTS AND DISCUSSION

For the simulation task of this work, we consider the scenario of massive MIMO communications where an N element transmit antenna BS is communicating through a Rayleigh channel with prior knowledge of the respective channel correlation matrix $\mathbf{R}_k$. The correlation matrices are based on correlation coefficient ρ such that $\mathbf{R}_{i,j} = \rho^{i-j}$ and $0 \le \rho \le 1$. The extreme values of ρ (0 and 1) show uncorrelated and fully correlated channel scenarios, respectively.

In Figure 3.2, the closed-form expression of OP is matched by with wide-ranging simulation means. We have considered mMIMO with $N = 128$, as well as a smaller diversity order of $N = 4$. We consider two cases of total users, namely, $K = 6$, and $K = 12$. Other parameters are set as $\sigma_k^2 = 10$ dBm, and $\rho = 0.15$. Now, for predefined threshold γ_{th}, the OP of a given user is directly proportional to the total number of cochannel interferes. It can be noted that, initially at the low value of γ_{th}, the OP is higher for a high number of transmit antennas, though this situation overturns as γ_{th} increases for both cases of users, namely, $K = 6$, and $K = 12$. A good degree of match exists between the analytical and the simulated results, thus validating the closed-form expressions.

Next in Figure 3.3, the impact of A on OP is shown by considering $N = 128$, and for $K = 4$, and $K = 12$. Now, for the whitened scenario, namely, $\rho = 0$, and for the fully correlated case, namely, $\rho = 1$, we convey the OP with respect to γ_{th} As per our prior observation, for lower γ_{th}, the OP is higher for the $\rho = 1$ case, however this pattern reverses with increasing value of γ_{th}.

Lastly, in Figure 3.4, the proposed optimization method is implemented using the MATLAB built-in optimization function "*fmincon*" via the "Sequential Quadratic Programming" method. The results show that the proposed method minimizes the

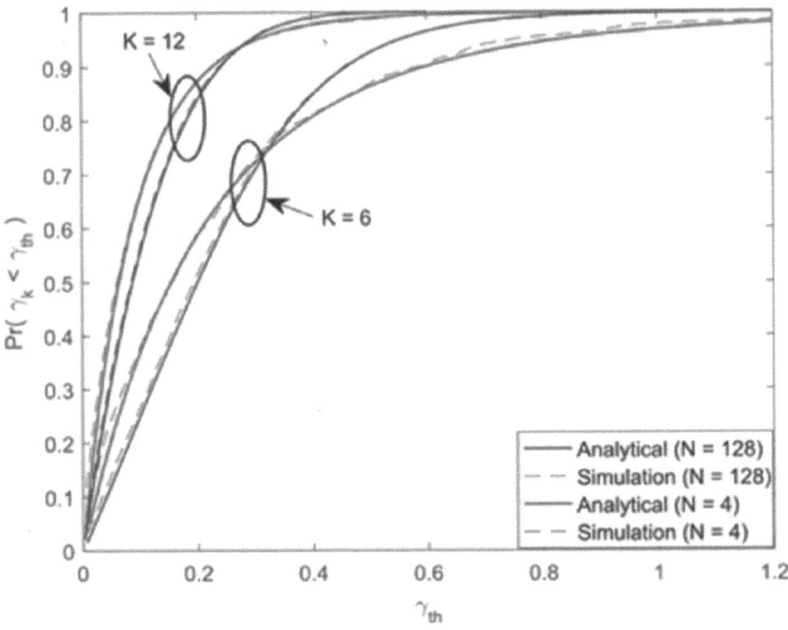

FIGURE 3.2   Effect of N and K on the OP [16].

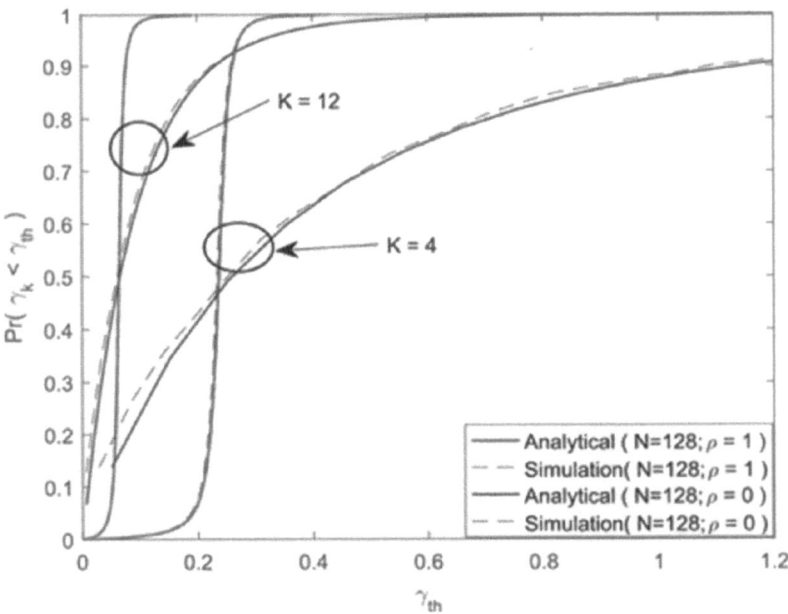

FIGURE 3.3   Impact of P and K on the OP for $N = 128$ [16].

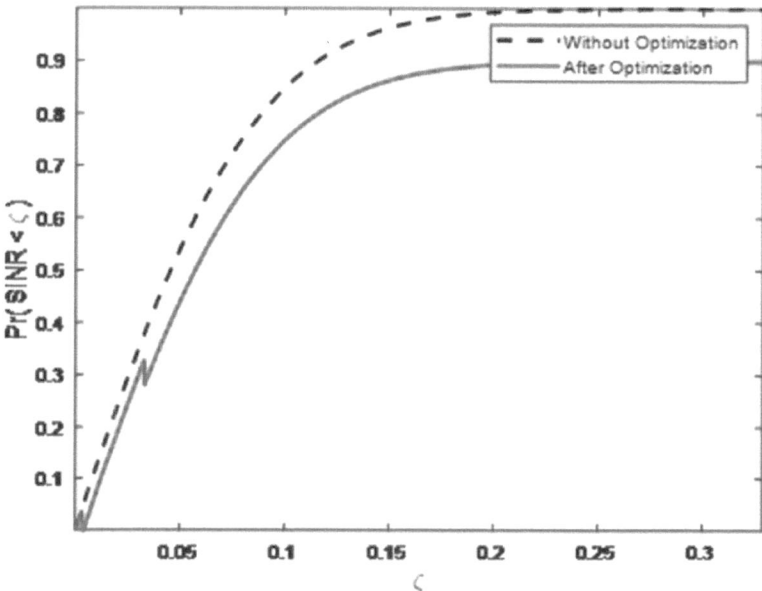

FIGURE 3.4   Result of beamforming optimization.

outage probability for all the threshold values showing improvement in the overall outage probability.

3.6   CONCLUSION

This chapter gave an exposition of recent works on the mMIMO downlink systems and presented a technique for achieving a closed-form analytical solution of OP for a statistical CSI based Rayleigh fading channel by employing an IQF approach. KPIs are examined by encompassing the impact of several system parameters.

REFERENCES

1. Marzetta, T. L. "Noncooperative cellular wireless with unlimited numbers of base station antennas," *IEEE Trans. Wireless Commun.*, vol. 9, no. 11, pp. 3590–3600, Nov. 2010.
2. Rusek, F. et al., "Scaling up MIMO: Opportunities and challenges with very large arrays," *IEEE Signal Process. Mag.*, vol. 30, pp. 40–46, Jan. 2013.
3. Cisco. Cisco Visual Networking Index: Global Mobile Data Traffic Forecast Update. [Online]. Available: www.cisco.com/c/en/us/solutions/collateral/executive-perspecti ves/annual-internet-report/white-paper-c11-741490.html
4. Lu, L. Li, G. Y. Swindlehurst, A. L. Ashikhmin, A. and Zhang, R. "An overview of massive MIMO: Benefits and challenges," *IEEE J. Sel.Topics Signal Process.*, vol. 8, no. 5, pp. 742–758, Oct. 2014.

5. Li, M. Lin, M. Zhu, W. P. Huang, Y. Nallanathan, A. and Yu, Q. "Performance analysis of MIMO MRC systems with feedback delay and channel estimation error," *IEEE Trans. Veh. Technol.*, vol. 65, no. 2, pp. 707–717, Feb. 2016.

6. van Chien, T. Björnson, E. and Larsson. E. G. (Jan. 2016). "Joint power allocation and user association optimization for massive MIMO systems." [Online]. Available: https://arxiv.org/abs/1601.02436

7. Björnson, E. Hoydis, J. Kountouris, M. and Debbah, M. "Massive MIMO systems with non-ideal hardware: Energy efficiency, estimation, and capacity limits," *IEEE Trans. Inf. Theory*, vol. 60, no. 11, pp. 7112–7139, Nov. 2014.

8. Zhang, X. Chen, F. and Wang, W. "Outage probability study of multiuser diversity in MIMO transmit antenna selection systems," *IEEE Signal Process. Lett.*, vol. 14, no. 3, pp. 161–164, Mar. 2007.

9. Zhou, Q. and Dai, H. "Asymptotic analysis on the interaction between spatial diversity and multiuser diversity in wireless networks," *IEEE Trans. Signal Process.*, vol. 55, no. 8, pp. 4271–4283, Aug. 2007.

10. Leadbetter, M. R. and Rootzen, H. "Extremal theory for stochastic processes," *Ann. Probab.*, vol. 16, pp. 431–478, Apr. 1988.

11. Al-Naffouri, T. Sharif, M. and Hassibi, B. "How much does transmit correlation affect the sum-rate scaling of MIMO Gaussian broadcast channels?" *IEEE Trans. Commun.*, vol. 57, no. 2, pp. 562–572, Feb. 2009.

12. Alouini, M. S. and Goldsmith, A. J. "Capacity of Rayleigh fading channels under different adaptive transmission and diversity-combining techniques," *IEEE Trans. Veh. Technol.*, vol. 48, no. 4, pp. 1165–1181, Jul. 1999.

13. Chiani, M. Win, M. Z. and Zanella, A. "On the capacity of spatially correlated MIMO Rayleigh-fading channels," *IEEE Trans. Inf. Theory*, vol. 49, no. 10, pp. 2363–2371, Oct. 2003.

14. Moinuddin, M. and Naseem, I. "A simple approach to evaluate the ergodic capacity and outage probability of correlated Rayleigh diversity channels with unequal signal-to-noise ratios," *EURASIP J. Wireless Commun. Netw.*, vol. 20, pp. 1–7, Dec. 2013.

15. Al-Naffouri, T. Y. Moinuddin, M. Ajeeb, N. Hassibi, B. and Moustakas, A. L. On the distribution of indefinite quadratic forms in Gaussian random variables," *IEEE Trans. Commun.*, vol. 64, no. 1, pp. 153–165, Jan. 2016.

16. Hassan, A. K. Moinuddin, M. Al-Saggaf, U. M. and Al-Naffouri, T. Y. Performance analysis of beamforming in MU-MIMO systems for Rayleigh fading channels. *IEEE Access*, 5, pp. 3709–3720, 2017.

17. Moinuddin, M. Al-Saggaf, U. M. and Hassan, A. K. King Abdulaziz University, Processing blind beamforming for multi-user multiple-input multiple-output (MU-MIMO) systems. U.S. Patent 11,252,045, 2022.

18. Hassan, A. K. Moinuddin, M. Al-Saggaf, U. M. Aldayel, O. Davidson, T. N. and Al-Naffouri, T. Y. Performance Analysis and Joint Statistical Beamformer Design for Multi-User MIMO Systems. *IEEE Commun. Let.*, vol. 24, no. 10, pp. 2152–6. Oct. 2020. doi: 10.1109/LCOMM.2020.3001556

4 5G Enabled Network Technology Trends for Smart Healthcare Systems

Satyanand Singh

CONTENTS

4.1   INTRODUCTION

Smart healthcare allows innovative medical software to provide patients with advanced medication and smart healthcare devices to increase the quality of healthcare by delivering real-time data for vital signs [1]. The aim of smart healthcare is to make it easier for patients to be provided with knowledge about medical conditions and their solutions. In the event of critical situations, smart healthcare encourages patients to take effective measures [2]. It helps remote check-up services by making use of 5G to minimize spending on medication and supports healthcare providers in the expansion of their services without geographical limits [3]. With the growth of smart cities, a comprehensive smart healthcare infrastructure is needed to ensure that people access health services. Owing to the massive population growth, conventional healthcare is unable to meet the needs of everybody. Health facilities are not available or affordable to all, despite providing an exemplary infrastructure and cutting-edge technology. One of the aims of smart healthcare is to assist consumers by educating them about any medical conditions and by keeping them aware of their health. Smart healthcare

DOI: 10.1201/9781003368311-4

empowers users to handle potential emergency conditions on their own [3]. It puts a focus on enhancing the user's quality and experience. Smart healthcare helps to use the services available to their full extent.

In general, connected health refers to any digital healthcare solution that can function remotely, with additional continuous health monitoring elements, emergency detection, and alarm capabilities [4]. Connected health focuses primarily on the goal of enhancing healthcare quality and productivity by allowing self-care and by complementing it with remote care. It has emerged in the telemedicine era, with users educated about their health, and feedback provided whenever possible [5]. Although smart healthcare refers to solutions that can function entirely independently, connected healthcare provides interventions that provide clinicians with input from patients. The broad classification of the smart healthcare industry, based on services, medical equipment, products used, applications, system management, and end-users is shown in Figure 4.1. In extending the uses for which the healthcare system is built, 5G communication technologies will play a vital role [6]. The successful integration of small devices through wireless technologies will help to introduce IoT remote health monitoring [2].

In the field of smart healthcare, 5G wireless communication systems and the IoT are transforming various applications such as asset management, behavioral change monitoring, remote monitoring, treatment compliance monitoring, life support, smarter medicine, telemedicine, and so forth. These applications will play an important role in the smart healthcare industry in the near future. By 2020, the smart

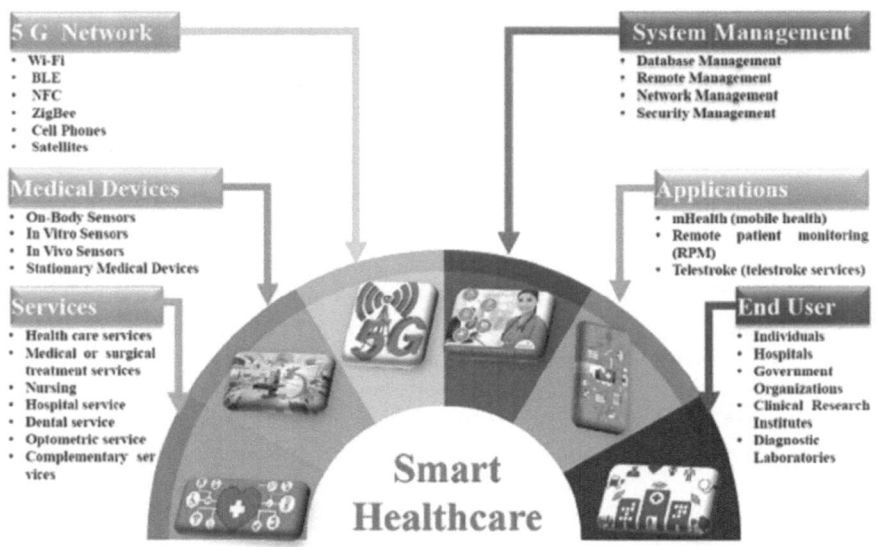

FIGURE 4.1 The broad classification of the smart healthcare industry based on services, medical equipment, products used, applications, system management, and end-users.

healthcare and IoT will reach approximately 117 billion US\$ across the industry [7]. Several technologies will be incorporated with the help of 5G wireless communication system to enable smart healthcare system [8]. A portable health app for checking pressure ulcers is recommended to record data electronically. In [9], it is proposed to use a smart healthcare application for evaluation and dietary checks. In [10], the author proposed a new strategy for mobile health applications. In [11], a wearable solution that supports mobility is proposed for the living environment. In [12], IoT applications based on mobile gateways is introduced for intelligent assistance in the mobile health environment. In [13], the IoT is considered a necessary element for medical use on electronic medical platforms. In [14], a wearable device is proposed to check the health of a wireless network consisting of sensors.

Smart antennas play an important role in 5G network communications [15]. Smart antennas use many important innovations to improve 5G coverage and capacity [16]. Beamforming (that is, vertical and horizontal) is one of the innovations, where RF energy is precisely focused on the contracted beam rather than radiating the same energy over a large area [17]. Beamforming is especially valuable for 5G NR. This is because the higher the millimeter wave RF, the more the loss of authentication and distance caused by the impact of obstructions (vehicle, building, and the like.) can be attenuated [18]. A more tuned beam of radio frequency energy helps ensure ideal transmission capacity and a higher probability of good signal quality [19]. However, it should be noted that the positioning line is still a problem, as the points of interest for beamforming decrease with attenuation [20].

4.2   CAPABILITIES AND CHALLENGES OF 5G TO ENHANCE FUTURE HEALTHCARE SYSTEMS

Network security and data privacy are critical to maximizing the potential of 5G networks in the healthcare sector [21]. Nothing is more sensitive than personal medical records [22]. An advanced communication program for healthcare interactions and activities is the foundation for patients to participate in the healthcare chains without worrying about data theft. Smart healthcare applications need to protect their 5G networks from network intruders [23]. Experts believe that in 5G networks used in healthcare there are three aspects that make powerful and effective network security and effective privacy strategy [24].

4.2.1   ZERO TRUST APPROACH

Reliable security measures must be implemented end-to-end for all devices and software on 5G networks [25]. Experts should assess the network risk of each device and application and grant access to network resources only if they meet high security standards. In addition, all software should be checked frequently for vulnerabilities and malware. Access to the most sensitive patient data should be reserved for a limited number of communication nodes, and these connections should be rigorously tested to check for potential security vulnerabilities [26].

4.2.2 Universal Code

Telecommunication service providers and other 5G user members should implement robust techniques of encryption in network traffic between end-users and operators to minimize the potential for data breaches and damage. As requirements and risks change, these techniques should be versatile enough to be gradually strengthened over time. The techniques also to be agile enough to prevent man-in-the-middle attacks where, for example, a hacker might eavesdrop on the communication between the service providers who were transferring data using 5G.

4.2.3 AI Orchestration

Machine learning (ML) and artificial intelligence AI need to play key roles in classifying and moderating various cyber risks and in producing a high-level of smart decision making to manage and eliminate network-security threats [27]. With the expansion of 5G in the healthcare sector, government regulators and policy makers need to create algorithms to guard the privacy of patients. The ML and AI algorithms may be used for the analysis of telecommunication network-traffic, data packet inspection, risk analysis, and the isolation of network attacks [28].

With the expansion of 5G in the healthcare sector, government regulators and policy makers have to make systems intelligent in order to protect the privacy of patients. These measures should be aimed at providing interoperability and extending telecommunications systems, applications, programs, and electronic system whilst safeguarding doctor to patient data security and the privacy of medical data. Doctor to patient medical equipment, medical data computation devices, and communication networks must have strict privacy to provide patient control over the medical data generation, store, and transmission by 5G-powered devices [29]. 5G onsite-enabled use situations in smart healthcare system and their capabilities are shown in Table 4.1.

In order to test for cyber security threats and confidentiality weaknesses in real-world smart healthcare use cases, it is necessary to establish parameters for testing all new devices and software.

In addition, data security testing and approval systems for technologies under development (cloud, AI, sensors, IoT, and so forth) need to be revised regularly to prevent privacy gaps in their development. Platforms and equipment [30].

A key pillar of smart healthcare is expected to be machine-to-machine (M2M) connectivity over 5G networks and the IoT [31]. The proposed strategy faces two major obstacles [32]. The first is that many terminals have established ultra-dense networks (for example, around 10^6 connections per square kilometer). The solutions needed to solve ultra-dense and scalability issues are suitable for IoT and M2M applications [33]. The second obstacle is that energy consumption based on the IoT depends on the application of the wireless sensor network, for example, the minimum battery life required under certain circumstances is 10 years [34]. Research on 5G deployment and commercialization began in 2014 and is expected to be completed by 2020 [35]. In addition to densifying networks and supporting a large number of IoT devices, 5G networks are expected to offer higher data rates. 5G networks not only have high data rates, but also other requirements such as large-scale connectivity, high-density

TABLE 4.1
5G Onsite-Enabled Use Cases in Smart Healthcare System

Use Case	Low Latency	High Bandwidth	Mobility	Reliability & Security	Capacity
Connected Ambulance	✓	✓	✓	✓	
HD virtual consultations		✓	✓	✓	
Remote patient monitoring			✓	✓	✓
Video-enabled medication adherence		✓		✓	
AR/VR assistance for the blind	✓	✓	✓	✓	
Distraction and rehabilitative therapy	✓	✓			
Remote expert for collaboration therapy	✓	✓		✓	
AR/VR for training and education	✓	✓		✓	
Real time high throughput computation	✓	✓	✓		
Video analytics for behavioral recognition	✓	✓		✓	

deployment, reliability, low latency, high energy efficiency, and long-distance communication to support IoT-based activity. They are designed to be flexible and versatile to support new applications in need smart healthcare applications.

This is the world of 5G broadband technology. Built-in processing intelligence allows you to manage your smart healthcare data so efficiently that it offers speeds in excess of 100 megabits/second, more data bandwidth, and less latency. This new 5G era integrates more networks, cloud-based storage, and a variety of linked devices and services. Extensive computing capabilities and virtual system architectures allow smart healthcare systems to open the Mobile Internet of Things (MIoT) [25]. Advanced digital networks integrate frameworks that connect billions of devices and sensors to drive advances in healthcare, education, resource management, transportation, agriculture, and many other areas. Much smart healthcare is underway today, but by soon it is expected to make great strides. Korean mobile operators can provide Internet services at super high speeds of 20 GB per second [36]. Other developed countries plan to offer 5G commercial networks by as early as possible. Most parts of the world are connected 24 hours a day, 7 days a week, and the number of digital devices is expected to grow dramatically. In the near future, consumers and businesses will establish a more immersive relationship with digital devices, which will enable them to receive quality medical care in real time at an affordable price. In the 5G world, distributed and independent computing devices will disappear, but real-time healthcare services will become the norm. This allows patients to get closer to the concept of digital fusion in science fiction than ever before.

5G is more than just an extension of 3G and 4G. On the contrary, heterogeneous networks that combine 4G, Wi-Fi, millimeter-wave and other wireless communication technologies are a transformative ecosystem. It combines cloud infrastructure, virtualized network cores, intelligent edge services, and derived distributed computing models with insights derived from data generated by billions of devices. 5G transforms the user-centered world into using large machine communications, transforming networks from enabling millions of devices into billions of connected devices that can intelligently execute information and perform intelligent commercialization. Emerging networks take advantage of different interfaces between authorization, authorization sharing, and the licensing of the low, medium, and high frequency spectrum. Not only does it increase capacity by design, but it also allows you to perform advanced signal processing on even the smallest devices and quickly connect to the processing power of the entire system.

It is important to remember that 5G uses an end-to-end device that moves communications to the network for computation [37]. 5G reflects the evolution from point-to-point systems that operate with the processing platforms needed to detect data from billions of devices and seamlessly sends these information packets to the right devices. Digital monitoring and prevention, AI diagnostics, AI-based therapy decisions, and digital therapy technologies will have a significant impact on the smart healthcare business as shown in Figure 4.2.

There are four aspects that make 5G different from its predecessor. These are connected devices, fast and intelligent networks, back-end services, and very low latency [38]. These qualities allow the world to be fully connected and interactive with different applications. This includes improved mobile broadband,

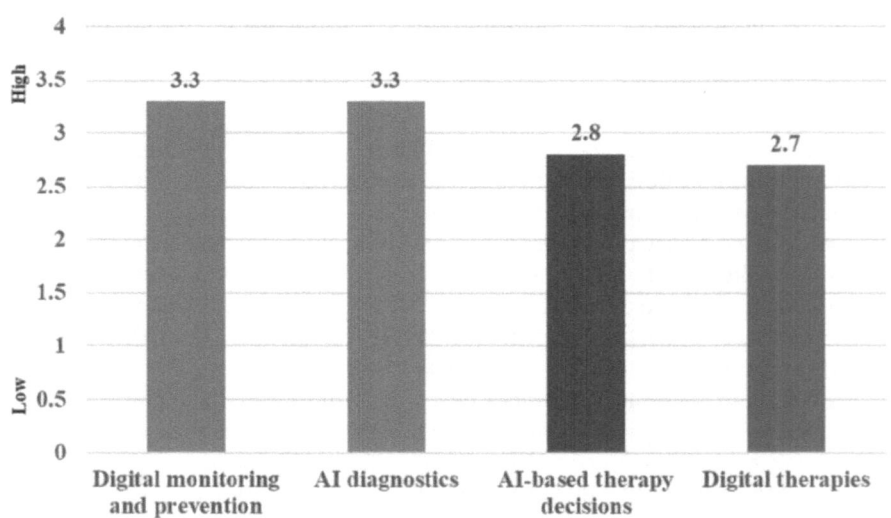

FIGURE 4.2 Potential application of digital monitoring and prevention, AI diagnostics, AI-based therapy decisions, digital therapy technologies in smart healthcare.

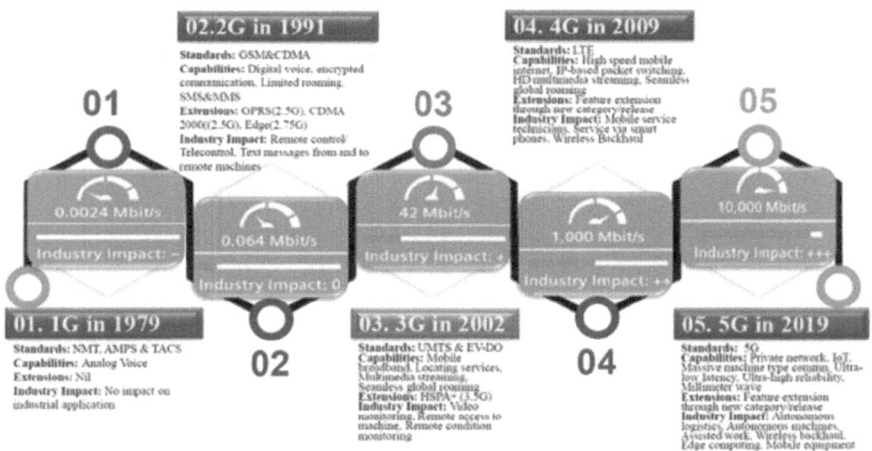

FIGURE 4.3 The evolution of wireless generations and their standards, capabilities, extensions, and industrial impacts.

machine-to-machine communication, AI, and advanced digital services. The evolution of wireless generations and their standards, capabilities, extension, and industrial impacts is shown in Figure 4.3.

4.3 5G ROLE IN REMOTE HEALTHCARE POTENTIALS

The 5G potential derives from its practical characteristics, which signify a major change from its 4G prototype. 5G is about 100 times faster than 4G and can handle more connections. The time it takes for an ultra-low latency network to process a request reinforces these benefits [39].

Controlling expectations is important when assessing the potential impact of 5G on healthcare. There is still some way to go for the widespread implementation of 5G [40]. There are 5G installations provided by all the largest country/region carriers, but their accessibility is usually inadequate for minor cells in city areas.

The large-scale expansion is expected in the year 2025 in many developed markets. In addition, the COVID-19 epidemic may have accelerated this timeline significantly, but it is unlikely that 5G applications such as wearable medical devices and telemedicine will be widely accepted by consumers in the coming years.

With the increasing need for confidentiality and reliability of medical data, people are beginning to raise concerns about security and privacy as medical records are transmitted over huge, often global public networks [41]. An eco-system that describes 5G integrated smart healthcare with the patient at the center of all activities, services, devices, and products is shown in Figure 4.4. In the situation of the latest COVID-19 pandemic, healthcare industries have paid great attention to the potential of 5G in supporting telemedicine services and computer-based physician consultation. This is useful if you need physical distance or if the patient is far away from the medical facility.

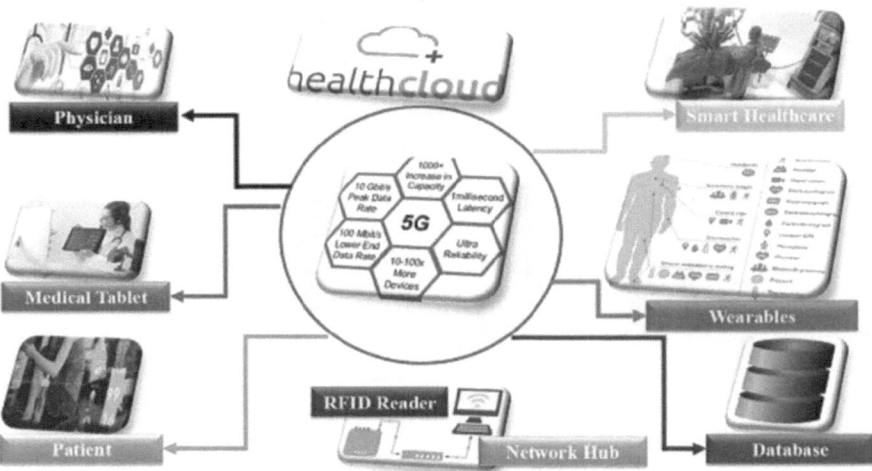

FIGURE 4.4 5G integrated smart healthcare with the patient at the center of all activities, services, devices, and products.

Existing 4G and fixed broadband infrastructure enables basic one-to-one low-touch conversations. However, 5G has great potential to facilitate these interactions [42]. For example, add sensors and virtual reality to a conference call to allow healthcare staff to monitor remotely vital parameters of a patient once the call is live. In addition, 5G can send large numbers of data packets, so smart healthcare can use a cloud-connected scanner to test changes in a patient's heart rate, sugar level in blood, and blood pressure, multiple times a day. These advances, in turn, provide more insight into the patient's routine medical care. With the addition of 5G and many other cutting-edge innovations, artificial intelligence, the IoT, health cloud, big data analytics, geolocation sensors, running screens, as well as various areas such as transportation, assembly, and retail [43]. It is integrated as a basic component of smart healthcare applications [44].

4.4 THE AI AND ML IMPACT ON SMART HEALTHCARE SYSTEMS DRIVEN BY 5G

The smart healthcare industry is a recession-resistant industry. Humans are in constant need of healthcare, so the healthcare industry can maintain its position in times of economic collapse and financial hardship. In fact, during the great depression in the United States, the healthcare industry expanded and added 852,000 jobs when the economy faced a severe slowdown. By 2021, the value of US healthcare AI is expected to reach $6.6 billion [45]. From clinical trials to new drug research and development, innovative medical devices, nanoparticles, AI, and machine learning technologies, all have the ability to touch and completely change all aspects. In fact, according to Accenture's research, applying AI to healthcare could save US $150 billion worldwide by 2026 [46]. The possibilities are endless. If AI is utilized correctly, then results will be unimaginable.

This problem, which has plagued the world for many years, is a triangle aimed at solving the basic health problem of high quality, low cost, and accessible treatment. Healthcare costs are usually high, so providing all three functions at the same time is a major healthcare challenge. The problem is that if you try to improve one element, you lose another. However, AI and 5G will be able to solve this problem in the near future by improving the current healthcare cost structure without breaking the triangle [47]. The key to this is 5G enabled AI machines, which patients can use for self-treatment in most cases, significantly reducing treatment costs by reducing contact with people and improving quality of life [48]. 5G driven AI and machine learning impact on the smart healthcare system is shown in Figure 4.5.

This is followed by using advanced analytics and machine learning techniques to unleash important insights from the billions of data elements associated with robot-assisted surgery [49]. When used properly, it can help overcome the associated inefficiencies and improve patient health. AI helps surgeons make better clinical decisions in real time during surgery and understand patient dynamics, especially during complex surgery [50–51]. In addition, the length of hospital stay for patients has been reduced by 21%. This ultimately reflects on the patient's postoperative care and long-term health. It also prevents patients from being hospitalized again, saving millions of dollars each year.

By 2026, AI-powered virtual nurses could ultimately save $20 billion annually in the U.S. healthcare industry [46]. They can answer patient questions 24 hours a day, 7 days a week, monitor patients and guide them as required. Currently, they act as a bridge for information exchange between caregivers (doctors) and care recipients (patients), determining which medications to start using, current health status, and the latest test results. The patient can be saved from many physical examinations

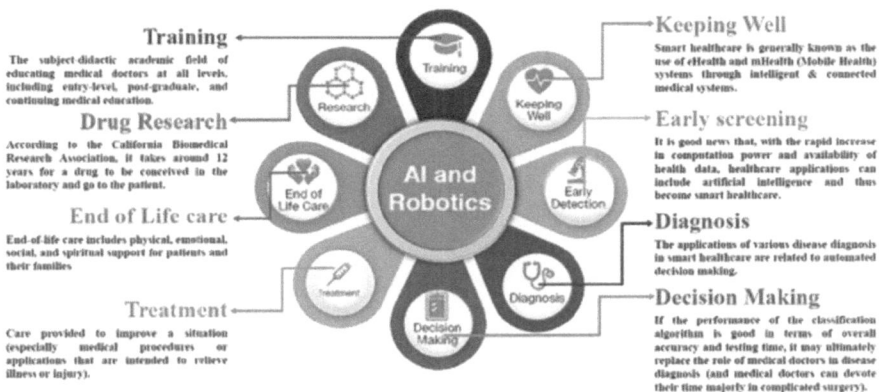

FIGURE 4.5 5G driven artificial intelligence and machine learning impact on the smart healthcare system.

by doctors, and high hospitalization rates can be prevented through simple, fun, and intelligent care. Care Angel is one of the best virtual nurses around. In addition to all the above features, smart healthcare can also have voice interactive and AI health checks.

4.5 FUTURE NEW HEALTHCARE ECOSYSTEMS WITH 5G

As the use of 5G in healthcare continues to grow, new interconnected healthcare ecosystems will begin to form as robotics, the IoT, and AI develop to accelerate application development [52]. It is believed that this ecosystem is in line with a relatively new idea, called 4P medicine: predictive, preventative, personal, and participatory [53].

Predictive: The new health ecosystem, combined with information on lifestyle and social factors, provides continuous real-time data on patient vital signs and associated alarms, enabling more accurate prediction of patient risk. At the same time, it provides healthcare providers with early warning about patient problems. Doctors and health care professional may utilize these visions to effectively to resolve problems earlier they escalate. 5G itself is not important in the forecasting process, but it supports the universal telecommunication interconnectivity and scale up of the healthcare ecosystem that can be used to collect, analyze, and share data.

Preventative: Being predictive can improve the ability of the general public to take precautionary measures. Fiji (Care Fiji App) is one example, and especially when COVID-19 occurred, this smartphone app was used to track the location and surrounding environment of a large number of people with unprecedented accuracy [54–55]. During a pandemic, this geographic information can combine with symptom profiles and continuous test reports to see who is at high risk, who can accidentally bring asymptomatic illness to others, and more. You can analyze the factors, and you can then notify high risk individuals by giving message alerts and medication to limit the fast progress of the pandemic.

Personal: The grouping of continuous online health monitoring of patients via 5G telecommunication networks offers many options to personalize common healthcare practices and involvements [56]. For example, healthcare service industries can utilize the tactile internet to remotely check patients (especially conditions) who are unable to reach large clinical facilities. In addition, health advice can be coordinated and confidentially provided to individuals in all populations [57–58].

Participatory: In the health ecosystem that supports 5G, patients become less involved with the operation of the healthcare system and are more involved in driving the outcome. Today, on average, patients in the United States spend 15 hours/year of their time with a healthcare professional and spend around five thousand hours taking care of themself when they wake up. Through these 5,000 hours of specific "activation" (namely, taking independent action to manage health, diagnosis, and treatment), patients can reduce the overall cost of the healthcare provider's healthcare systems. It is believed that this can improve the quality of life and health care of the general public. According to one study, after managing demographics and health, the cost of active patients was reduced by $1,987 annually. This was a 31% reduction compared to inactive patients.

4.6 PERSONALIZED HEALTHCARE SYSTEM: ROLES OF 5G

The introduction of 5G in the first phase of 2020 heralded future healthcare transformation with fast response times and short latency. 5G facilitates the development of patient personalization, including continuous monitoring of each patient's daily health through the Internet of Medical Things (IoMT), wearable devices, remote diagnostics and healthcare delivery [59–60]. With virtual reality (VR) and augmented reality (AR) home digital therapy is supported. Unleash AI/ML into big data to optimize healthcare diagnostics and insights [61]. Figure 4.6 shows a 5G integrated personalized healthcare system with predictive, preventative, personal, and participation values [62].

4.7 CONCLUSION

5G offers more applications and more remarkable benefits, and there is no better inducement to offer more comprehensive portable healthcare services. Despite the enormous costs of innovation, smart healthcare services can still generate revenue for local emergency clinics and at the same time require a large amount of patient investment funding. Smart healthcare systems and digital health applications have the potential to change current healthcare service processes. With the advent of 5G, further management and policy settings need to be considered to address issues such

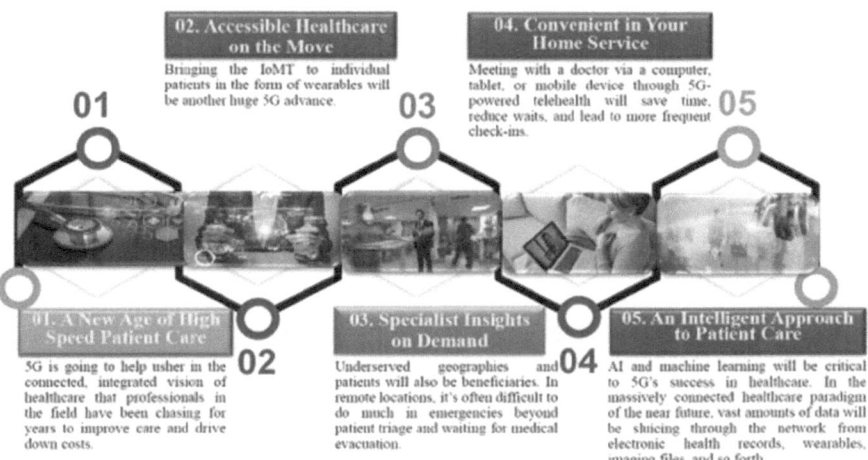

FIGURE 4.6 5G integrated personalized healthcare system with predictive, preventative, personal, and participatory values.

as welfare and protection. There is an urgent need for an appropriate environment to spread the benefits of 5G to customers, organizations, and society, and a strong governance structure and appropriate guidelines are essential.

5G can significantly advance healthcare, patient service, treatment, and healthcare programs by transforming healthcare and providing reliability, speed, and scalability for networks. But with the recent emergence of new ideas surrounding this topic, healthcare companies and healthcare providers should be particularly interested, especially when pandemics remind us of the incompetence and vulnerabilities of healthcare systems in the face of natural disasters. There is the belief that testing 5G applications will determine if any of the three main benefits of these telecommunication networks (ultra-fast broadband, ultra-low latency, large machine connectivity) will be significantly improved. Overall, the information is clear. Combining 5G with other key technologies can create opportunities to change many aspects of patient care while facilitating new healthcare ecosystems that are more closely linked (and with resources) than existing systems, that are smarter and more efficient. There are still many obstacles that need to be overcome in terms of institutions, culture, and technology before 5G networks become commonplace in healthcare.

REFERENCES

1. Soldani, D. C. D., Fadini, F., Rasanen, H., Duran, J., Niemela, T., Hoglund, N., N. T., Doppler, K., Himanen, T., and Laiho, J. "5G mobile systems for healthcare," in *IEEE 85th Vehicular Technology Conference (VTC Spring), Sydney, NSW, Australia*, pp. 1–5, 2017.
2. Sundaravadivel, M. K., Kougianos, P., Mohanty, E., Ganapathiraju, S. P., "Everything You Wanted to Know about Smart Health Care: Evaluating the Different Technologies and Components of the Internet of Things for Better Health," *IEEE Consum. Electron. Mag.*, vol. 7, no. 1, pp. 18–28, 2018.
3. Mohanty, B. S. P., Choppali, U., and Kougianos, E. "Everything you about smart cities," *IEEE Consum. Electron. Mag.*, vol. 5, no. 3, pp. 60–70, 2016.
4. Liu, W., Jia, X., Zhang, M., and Lu, X. "A novel multichannel Internet of things based on dynamic spectrum sharing in 5G communication," *IEEE Internet Things J.*, vol. 6, pp. 5962–5970, 2018.
5. Brito, J. M. "Technological Trends for 5G Networks Influence of E-Health and IoT Applications," *Int. J. Heal. Med Commun.*, vol. 9, pp. 1–22, 2018.
6. Li, D. "5G and intelligence medicine—How the next generation of wireless technology will reconstruct healthcare?" *Precis. Clin. Med.*, vol. 2, pp. 205–208, 2019.
7. McCue, T. "$117 billion market for the internet of things in healthcare by 2020," *Forbes Tech.* 2015.
8. Parchin, R., and Abd-Alhameed, N. O. "A compact Vivaldi antenna array for 5G channel sounding applications," in *Proceedings of the 12th European Conference on Antennas and Propagation (EuCAP 2018), London, UK*, pp. 9–13, 2018.
9. Rodrigues, I., Lopes, J. J., Silva, I. M., and Torre, B. M. "A new mobile ubiquitous computing application to control obesity: SapoFit," *Informatics Heal. Soc. Care*, vol. 38, pp. 37–53, 2013.
10. Silva, L., Rodrigues, B. M., Lopes, J. J., Machado, I. M., and Zhou, T. M. "A novel cooperation strategy for mobile health applications," *IEEE J. Sel. Areas Commun*, vol. 31, no. 28–36, 2013.

11. Yang, K., Urke, G., and Øvsthus, A. R. "Mobility Support of IoT Solution in Home Care Wireless Sensor Network," in *2018 Ubiquitous Positioning, Indoor Navigation and Location-Based Services (UPINLBS),Wuhan, China, 22–23 March*, pp. 75–480, 2018.

12. Santos, V., Rodrigues, J., Silva, J. J., Casal, B. M., Saleem, J., and Denisov, K. "An IoT-based mobile gateway for intelligent personal assistants on mobile health environments," *J. Netw. Comput. Appl.*, vol. 71, pp. 194–204, 2016.

13. Vilela, V., Rodrigues, P. H., Solic, J. J., Saleem, P., and Furtado, K. "Performance evaluation of a Fog-assisted IoT solution for e-Health applications," *Futur. Gener. Comput. Syst.*, vol. 97, pp. 379–386, 2019.

14. Ahad, N., Al Faisal, A., Ali, S., Jan F., and Ullah, B. "Design and Performance Analysis of DSS (Dual Sink Based Scheme) Protocol for WBASNs," *Adv. Remote Sens.*, vol. 6, pp. 249–259, 2017.

15. Parchin, N. O., Basherlou, H. J., Al-Yasir, Y. I., Abd-Alhameed, R. A., Abdulkhaleq, A. M., and Noras, J. M. "Recent developments of reconfigurable antennas for current and future wireless communication systems," *Electronics*, vol. 8, no. 2, pp. 1–17, 2019.

16. Parchin, N. O., Alibakhshikenari, M., Basherlou, H. J., Abd-Alhameed, R., Rodriguez, J., and Limiti, E. "MM-wave phased array quasi-Yagi antenna for the upcoming 5G cellular communications," *Appl. Sci.*, vol. 9, no. 5, pp. 1–14, 2019.

17. Mohammad, L., Virdee, A., See, B. S., Abd-Alhameed, C. H., Falcone, R. A., and Ernesto, F. "High-Gain Metasurface in polyimide on-chip Antenna Based on cRLH-tL for Sub-terahertz integrated circuits," *Sci. Rep.*, vol. 10, no. 4298, pp. 1–9, 2020.

18. Saeidi-Manesh, G., and Zhang, H. "Low cross-polarization, high-isolation microstrip patch antenna array for multi-mission applications," *IEEE Access*, vol. 7, pp. 5026–5033, 2018.

19. Saeidi-Manesh, G., and Zhang, H. "Challenges and Limitations of the Cross-Polarization Suppression in Dual-Polarization Antenna Arrays using Identical Subarrays," *IEEE Trans. Antennas Propag.*, vol. 68, no. 4, pp. 2853–2866, 2019.

20. Alibakhshikenari, E., Virdee, M., Shukla, B. S., See, P., Abd-Alhameed, C. H., Khalily, R., Falcone, M., and Limiti, F. "Antenna mutual coupling suppression over wideband using embedded periphery slot for antenna arrays," *Electronics*, vol. 7, no. 9, pp. 1–11, 2018.

21. Scott, M. "What 5G Will Mean for You," *New York Times*.

22. Osseiran, M. et al, "Scenarios for 5G mobile and wireless communications: The vision of the METIS project," *IEEE Commun. Mag*, vol. 52, no. 5, pp. 26–35, 2014.

23. Palacios, J. W. J., Bielsa, G., and Casari, P. "Single-and multiple-access point indoor localization for millimeter-wave networks," *IEEE Trans. Wirel. Commun.*, vol. 18, no. 3, pp. 1927–1942, 2019.

24. Hall, D. M. J. L. "For telehealth to succeed privacy and security risks must be identified and addressed," *Heal. Aff.*, vol. 33, no. 2, pp. 216–221, 2014.

25. King, I. "5G Networks Will Do Much More Than Stream Better Cat Videos," *Bloomberg News.* 2016.

26. Naik, G. P. B. N., Gupta, R., Singh, A., and Soni, S. L. "Realtime smart patient monitoring and assessment amid COVID19 pandemic–an alternative approach to remote monitoring," *J. Med. Syst.*, vol. 44, no. 7, pp. 1–2, 2020.

27. Singh, B. "Best Practices for Orchestrating AI Solutions," *Global Head of Digital Transformation*, pp. 1–9.

28. Semantha, B. S. F. H., Azam, S., and Yeo, K. C. "A systematic literature review on privacy by design in the healthcare sector," *Electronics*, vol. 9, no. 3, p. 452, 2020.

29. Kemmer, N. C. F., Reich, C., and Knahl, M. "Software-defined privacy," in *2016 IEEE International Conference on Cloud Engineering Workshop (IC2EW), 2016*, pp. 25–29, 2016.

30. O'Connor, C. H. Y., Rowan, W., and Lynch, L. "Privacy by design: Informed consent and internet of things for smart health," in *Comput. Sci. 113*, pp. 653–658, 2017.

31. Agiwal, A., Saxena, M., and Roy, N. "Towards connected living: 5G enabled internet of things (IoT)," *IETE Tech. Rev*, vol. 36, pp. 190–202, 2019.

32. Andreev, S., Galinina, O., Pyattaev, A., Gerasimenko, M., Tirronen, T., and Torsner, J. "Understanding the IoT connectivity landscape: A contemporary m2m radio technology roadmap," *IEEE Commun. Mag.*, vol. 5, no. 39, 2015.

33. de Mattos, P. R. G. W. D. "M-health solutions using 5G networks and M2M communications," *IT Prof*, vol. 18, no. 3, pp. 24–29, 2016.

34. Palattella, L., Dohler, M. R., Grieco, M., Rizzo, A., Torsner, G., Engel, J., and Ladid, T. "Internet of things in the 5G era: Enablers, architecture, and business models," *IEEE J. Sel. Areas Commun.*, vol. 34, no. 3, pp. 510–527, 2016.

35. Chih-Lin, Z., Han, I., Xu, S., Sun, Z., and Pan, Q. "5G: Rethink mobile communications for 2020+," *Philos. Trans. R. Soc. A Math. Phys. Eng. Sci.*, vol. 374, no. 2062, pp. 2010–2020, 2016.

36. Torres, I. "20 GBs per second 5G Network to Make Debut in 2018 Winter Olympics." 2015.

37. Ahad, A., Tahir, A., Aman Sheikh, M., Ahmed, M., Mughees, K. I., and Numani, A. "Technologies trend towards 5G network for smart health-care using IoT: A review," *Sensors*, vol. 20, p. 4047, 2020.

38. Militano, A., Araniti, L., Condoluci, G., Farris, M., and Iera, I. "Device-to-device communications for 5G internet of things," *EAI Endorsed Trans. Internet Things*, vol. 1, pp. 1–15, 2015.

39. Kumar, A., Albreem, M. A., Gupta, M., Alsharif, M. H., and Kim, S. "Future 5G network based smart hospitals: Hybrid detection technique for latency improvement," *IEEE Access*, vol. 8, pp. 153240–153249, 2020, doi: 10.1109/ACCESS.2020.3017625.

40. Dhanvijay, S. C., and Patil, M. M. "Internet of things: A survey of enabling technologies in healthcare and its applications," *Comput. Networks*, vol. 153, pp. 113–131, 2019.

41. Rao, E. B. F. "Privacy techniques for edge computing systems," *IEEE*, vol. 107, pp. 1632–1654, 2019.

42. Kiah, M. H. M. M., Al-Bakri, S., Zaidan, A., and Zaidan, B. "Design and develop a video conferencing framework for realtime telemedicine applications using secure group-based communication architecture," *J. Med. Syst.*, vol. 38, no. 10, p. 133, 2014.

43. Goudos, S., Dallas, S., Chatziefthymiou, P., and Kyriazakos, S. "A survey of IoT key enabling and future technologies: 5G, mobile IoT, sematic web and applications," *Wirel. Pers. Commun.*, vol. 97, pp. 1645–1675, 2017.

44. Talal, O. A. M. et al, "Smart home-based IoT for real-time and secure remote health monitoring of triage and priority system using body sensors," *Multidriven Syst. Rev. J. Med. Syst.*, vol. 43, no. 2, p. 42, 2019.

45. Kumar, A., Dhanagopal, R., Albreem, M. A., and Le, D-N., "A comprehensive study on the role of advanced technologies in 5G based smart hospital," *Alex. Eng. J.*, vol. 60, no. 6, pp. 5527–5536, December 2021.

46. Matt Collier, L. Y., and P. C., and Fu, R. "Artificial Intelligence," *Healthcare's New Nervous System*, pp. 1–8, 2017.

47. Natarajan, P., and Frenzel, J. C. *Demystifying big data and machine learning for healthcare.* 2017.

48. Kumar, U. D., and Gandhi, P. M. "A novel three-tier internet of things architecture with machine learning algorithm for early detection of heart diseases," vol. 65, pp. 222–235, 2018.

49. Gupta, N. K. R., Tanwar, S., and Tyagi, S. "Tactile-internet based telesurgery system for healthcare 4.0: An architecture, research challenges, and future directions," *IEEE Netw.*, vol. 33, no. 6, pp. 22–29, 2019.

50. Fogel, J., and Kvedar, A. L. "Artificial intelligence powers digital medicine," *npj Digit. Med.*, vol. 1, no. 5, pp. 1–4, 2018.

51. Domingos, P. *The master algorithm: How the quest for the ultimate learning machine will remake our world.* Basic Books; 1st edition, 22 September 2015.

52. Porambage, T. T. P., Okwuibe, J., Liyanage, M., and Ylianttila, M. "Survey on multi-access edge computing for internet of things realization," *IEEE Commun. Surv. Tutor,* vol. 20, no. 4, pp. 2961–2991, 2018.

53. Singhal, S., Kayyali, B., Levin, R., and Greenberg, Z. "The next wave of healthcare innovation: The evolution of ecosystems," *Healthcare Systems & Services*, pp. 1–13, 2020. www.mckinsey.com/industries/healthcare-systems-and-services/our-insights/the-next-wave-of-healthcare-innovation-the-evolution-of-ecosystems

54. Albahri, A., and Hamid, R. A. "Role of biological data mining and machine learning techniques in detecting and diagnosing the novel Coronavirus (COVID-19):-A systematic review," *J. Med,* vol. 44, no. 7, p. 122, 2020.

55. Patrinley, M. K. J. R., Berkowitz, S.T., Zakria, D., Totten, D. J., and Drolet, B. C. "Lessons from operations management to combat the COVID-19 pandemic," *J. Med. Syst.*, vol. 44, no. 7, pp. 1–2, 2020.

56. Lee, L. C. W. Y., Loo, L. J., and Chuah, T. C. "Dynamic network slicing for multitenant heterogeneous cloud radio access networks," *IEEE Trans. Wirel. Commun.*, vol. 4, no. 18, pp. 2146–2161, 2017.

57. Hewa, M. L. T., Gür, G., Kalla, A., Ylianttila, M., and Bracken, A. "The Role of Blockchain in 6G: Challenges, Opportunities and Research Directions," in *2020 2nd 6G Wireless Summit (6G SUMMIT), Levi, Finland,* pp. 1–5, 2020.

58. Chandrasekaran, S., Bowen, C., Roscow, J., and Zhang, Y. "Micro-scale to nano-scale generators for energy harvesting: Self powered piezoelectric, triboelectric and hybrid devices," *Phys. Rep.*, vol. 792, pp. 1–33, 2019.

59. Japheth Worthy, M. S., Mehta, M., O'Driscoll, N., and Friberg, H. and J. "IRC Healthcare & Life Sciences Practice Group team," *Globally Connected*, pp. 1–10, 2020.

60. Amendola, G., Lodato, S., Manzari, R., Occhiuzzi, S., and Marrocco, C. "RFID technology for IoT-based personal healthcare in smart spaces," *IEEE Internet Things J.*, vol. 1, no. 2, pp. 144–152, 2014.

61. Saxena, M. "The Future of Healthcare: Data-Driven Personalized Medicine at Scale," *Forbes*, pp. 1–5, 2020.

62. Boccardi, P. P. F., Heath, R.W., Lozano, A., and Marzetta, T. L. "Five disruptive technology directions for 5G," *IEEE Commun. Mag*, vol. 52, no. 2, pp. 74–80, 2014.

5 Non-Orthogonal Multiple Access Transmission for 5G Technology
Practical Considerations

Ibrahim Almujtaba and Abdulah Aljohani

CONTENTS

5.1 INTRODUCTION

There are two methods for NOMA techniques. The two techniques are known as code domain and power domain [1]. To increase the users' detection and for the minimization of symbol error rates, the CD-NOMA uses random-Gaussian codes at the transmitter and compressive sensing on the receiving end. Moreover, because the transmitted signal is sparse, low-density spreading coding with CMDA (LDS-CDMA) and LDS-aided OFDM can be used (LDS-OFDM). In the power-domain NOMA (PD-NOMA), several user signals are jointly superimposed to utilize a

DOI: 10.1201/9781003368311-5

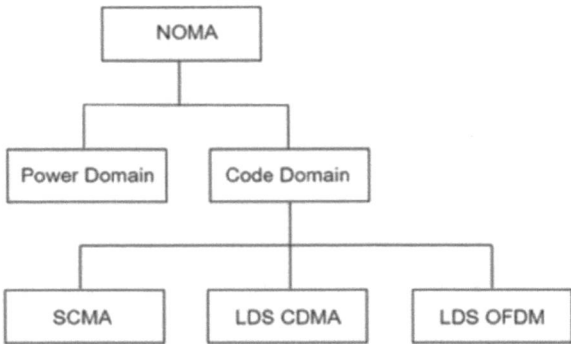

FIGURE 5.1   The main NOMA schemes classifications.

similar (frequency/time/code) resource by designating separate power-levels for each user. Likewise, dirty paper coding or SIC is used to decode the users' communication signals at the receiving end [2–3]. Figure 5.1 depicts the classifications of NOMA techniques.

In this chapter, we will discuss and analyze the two techniques used in NOMA, Firstly, we will analyze the power-domain NOMA (PD-NOMA) in a real life transmission scenario then we will analyze the code-domain NOMA (CD-NOMA) in the same scenario. A literature review will be presented in Section 5.3. While in Section 5.4, the proposed system model and its result will be discussed. Finally, our conclusion will be offered in Section 5.5.

5.2   OBJECTIVES

The main objectives of the chapter are as follow:

1.   To assess the PD-NOMA system's effectiveness and performance.
2.   To assess the CD-NOMA system's effectiveness and performance.
3.   To develop a realistic transmission scenario for downlink NOMA.

5.3   RELATED LITERATURE REVIEW

Enormous numbers of researchers have demonstrated that NOMA systems can fulfill the requirements of fifth generation (5G). For example, the PD-NOMA was analyzed when transmitting over a fading channel in [4], where it was shown that NOMA can increase spectral efficiency significantly when compared with OMA.

In [3], the researchers used a SIC receiver in a downlink-NOMA system, based on a projected future enhancement in device processing capabilities. They show that the downlink NOMA with the use of SIC operates well and improves cell-edge user throughput and overall capacity, based on system-level analyses [3].

Furthermore, the progress of NOMA is surveyed in [5] by the authors in 5G systems. The authors reviewed user fairness, power allocation techniques, capacity analysis and the user pairing method in NOMA. In addition, the authors identified the operationalization of NOMA with different methods of communication for example space time coding, cooperative communication, beam foaming, MIMO, and network coding.

In [6] the researchers, did comparison research of OMA and NOMA and found that a hybrid OMA/NOMA methodology could be a helpful solution for modern wireless cellular communications. Research in allocating power-efficient resources for multi-carrier (MC) NOMA was also undertaken in [7] with the goal of lowering total power usage. The study advocated low-complexity scheduling and sub-optimal power allocation for users. An overview of promising modulation scheme-aided NOMA is presented in [8], where the spectral efficiency, out-of-band leakage, and BER performances were examined. While in [9] a power allocation-aided beamforming is proposed for a downlink NOMA scenario, where a significant power reduction was exhibited, when compared to OMA systems.

In [10], the author investigated beamforming to decrease the transmitted power for the downlink 2-user MISO based NOMA system. They proposed a half- zero for-cing (ZF) technique which only reduces the interference from the cell-interior user signal. Meanwhile, SIC is used to remove the interference from the signal of the cell-edge user. A closed form expression for the beamforming vectors was derived under the half-ZF scheme. Compared with the conventional ZF method, the half-ZF can achieve lower power consumption.

A combination of power allocation and beamforming in a downlink MIMO multi-user system which employs NOMA is presented in [11]. The study addresses a scen-ario where they divide users into two groups by users' QoS, specifically, the users in the first group are expected to be served whereas the users in the second group were required to reach target rates on their own. The proposed method showed a significant sum rate improvement.

In [12], a multicast beamforming-aided superposition modulation (SPM) was investigated for multi-resolution broadcast. In the study, users' messages of low and high priorities were to be transmitted for the nearby user, while only a message of low priority is to be transmitted to a distant user. In [13], a multi-user NOMA beamforming problem was formulated as a semi-definite programming problem and generalized to include the conventional multi-user beamforming. The authors studied a low-complexity approach to decide successive interference cancellation sets for the generalized NOMA. They showed that their proposed method can have a better per-formance than the conventional BF.

In [14], to increase the sum capacity, the author suggested a NOMA based multi-user system of beam forming. The suggested method shared a beamforming vector for two users, which means that the supported number of users is increased. They additionally proposed an allocation of a power and clustering algorithm for the mini-mization of interference and to enhance the sum capacity.

In [15], NOMA with SIC in downlink multi-user MIMO cellular systems was investigated, at these points the quantity of antennas at the transmitter side were less than the quantity of receiver antennas. The proposed linear beamforming tech-nique highlighted that the capacity gain performance is significantly improved when compared with the MIMO-OMA counterpart. Finally, a comprehensive NOMA survey is offered in [16].

5.4 THE SYSTEM MODEL AND RESULTS

This part will be used to introduce the PD-NOMA, CD-NOMA, and the realistic transmission of a PD-NOMA, alongside with their corresponding results.

5.4.1 POWER-DOMAIN NOMA

The schematic of the overall PD-NOMA scheme is shown in Figure 5.2. The two users' signals, namely near user and far user will first be superimposed before the transmission. Below, each of the Figure 5.2 blocks will be explained further.

5.4.1.1 Superposition Modulation (SPM)

Superposition modulation (SPM) is a widely known technique for non-orthogonal schemes. The concept of superposition modulation was introduced first in [17], the SPM joins two messages and transmits them simultaneously by encoding them in one signal. A signaling scheme is characterized by a constellation and a mapping rule. These two concepts are used in SPM. The SPM constellation for joining two users in a single signal is shown in Figure 5.3.

At the transmitter side, the transmitted signals for the two users are superimposed using superposition coding (SC) as shown in Figure 5.4.

For example, the QPSK modulated signals S_1 and S_2 will be linearly combined to generate a 16-QAM X_{SPM} using SPM as follows:

$$X_{SPM} = r_1 s_1 + r_2 s_2 \qquad (5.1)$$

where r_1 and r_2 are scaling factors to protect the signals, where a signal with higher scaling factor will be more protected with the condition that $r_1 s_1 + r_2 s_2 = 1$.

5.4.1.2 Successive Interference Cancellation (SIC)

A typical MIMO system can be described by:

$$y = Hx + n \qquad (5.2)$$

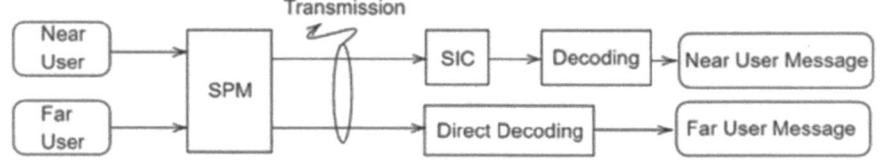

FIGURE 5.2 Power-Domain NOMA schematic diagram.

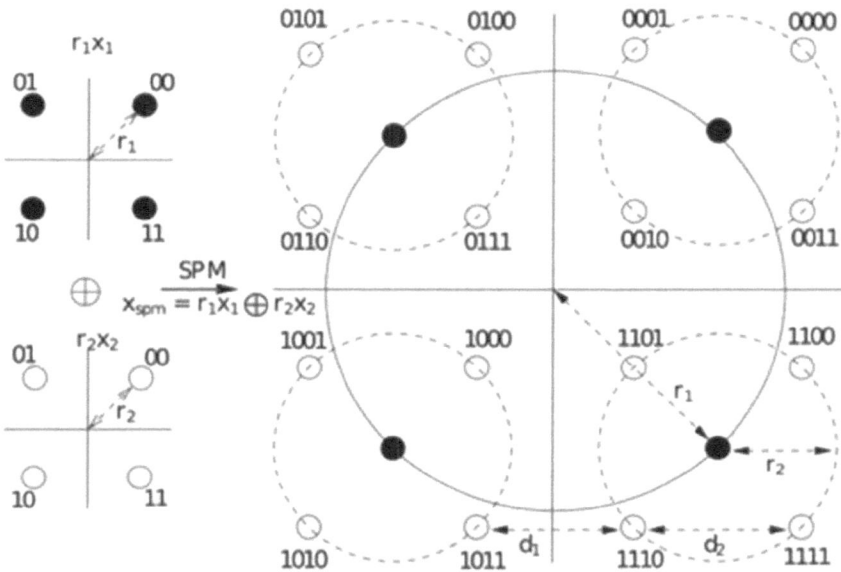

FIGURE 5.3 Constellation diagram explaining superposition coding for NOMA system.

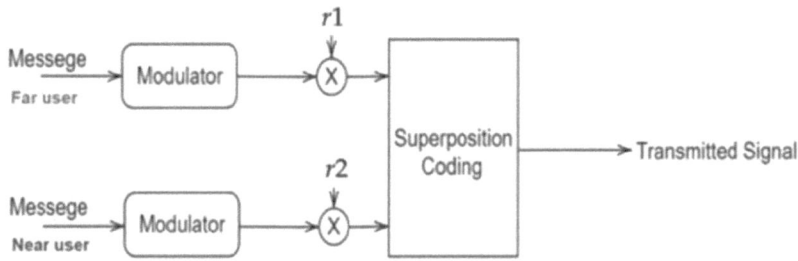

FIGURE 5.4 PD-NOMA transmitter.

where H is the channel, x is the transmitted signal, and n denotes the AWGN with mean zero and variance σ_N^2.

Two common receiver designs are minimum mean square error (MMSE) and zero-forcing (ZF) for the MIMO system [18]. The ZF detector only focuses on the elimination of channel effect and has the form of

$$w_{ZF} = H^H \left(HH^H\right)^{-1} \qquad (5.3)$$

where superscript "H" denotes the Hermitian transpose operation. The MMSE detector additionally considers the impact of additive noise, and improves the ZF detector with the form of

$$w_{MMSE} = H^H \left(HH^H + diag\left(\sigma_N^2\right) \right)^{-1} \qquad (5.4)$$

Since the MMSE detector also depresses the noise effect, it has a better performance than the ZF detector.

For the purpose of improving the performance of the MMSE detector in interference cancellation, the authors in [19], proposed a novel modification of it, resulting in the so-called MMSE interference rejection combining (MMSE-IRC) detector. It is worth mentioning that the complexity of linear detectors is often lower than that of nonlinear ones, and hence they are more commonly employed in the SIC technique. SIC will be performed by the user with low power allocated to it to cancel the effect of other user interference. The nearby user with less interference in the channel decodes and cancels the distant user's signal first then decodes its signal, while the distant user decodes its signal directly due to fading of the other user's signal and will not need the use of SIC in its condition. Figure 5.5, shows the flow chart of the codeword-level SIC that we used in our system.

In the receiver side, we only use SIC on the near user s_{near} because the far user s_{far} will decode directly because of the low power allocated to the near signal s_{near}. It is assumed that the signal will be faded and will not reach the far user s_{far}. The receiver system is shown in Figure 5.6.

The received signals at the two users are

$$z_{far} = gx + n_{far} = g\left(r_1 s_{far} + r_2 s_{near}\right) + n_{far}$$

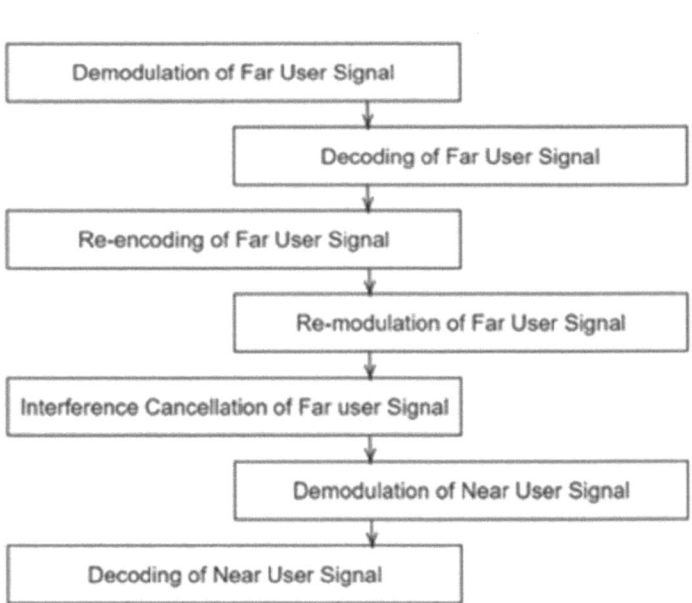

FIGURE 5.5 Flow chart for code word level SIC.

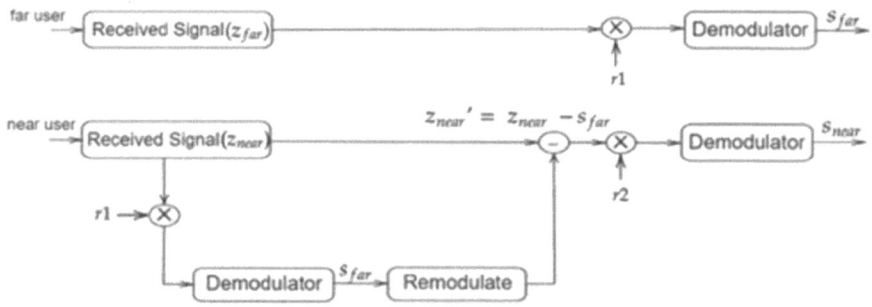

FIGURE 5.6   PD-NOMA receiver.

$$z_{near} = hx + n_{near} = h\left(r_1 s_{far} + r_2 s_{near}\right) + n_{near} \tag{5.5}$$

Where h and g represent Rayleigh channel vector which is zero mean complex circular Gaussian with co-variance matrix R_i for $i \in \{far, near\}$.

5.4.1.3   Simulation Results

The BER performance of the near user s_{near} and the far user s_{far} of the system is shown in Figure 5.7, with power allocated of P1 = 0.8 and P2 = 0.2. Note that each user uses binary phase shift keying modulation (BPSK), and the signals go through AWGN and Rayleigh fading channels. The PD-NOMA performance decreases with the increasing of number of users because the inter-user interference and the residual interference will increase due to the increasing of the SIC error.

The simulation result in Figure 5.7 shows the bit error rate for a PD-NOMA downlink system under a Rayleigh fading channel.

The simulation result in Figure 5.8 shows the performance of turbo coding in a NOMA system under a Rayleigh fading channel and saves 20 dB compared to the uncoded NOMA system.

5.4.2   Code-Domain NOMA

Figure 5.9 illustrates the overall schematic diagram of the CD-NOMA that will be tested. Each block is further explained below.

5.4.2.1   Sparse Code Multiple Access (SCMA)

SCMA [20], which is known as sparse code multiple access is one of the main methods of CD NOMA. The SCMA is a multi-dimensional code book non orthogonal spreading method. Likewise, the bits are immediately mapped by the SCMA encoder to multi-dimensional complicated code-words that have already been defined in a code–book set. An SCMA encoder is defined as a k-dimensional complicated codebook of size M that maps "$\log_2$ (M)" bits into it. The factor graph matrix is used to represent the collection of codebooks in the SCMA system. The message passing

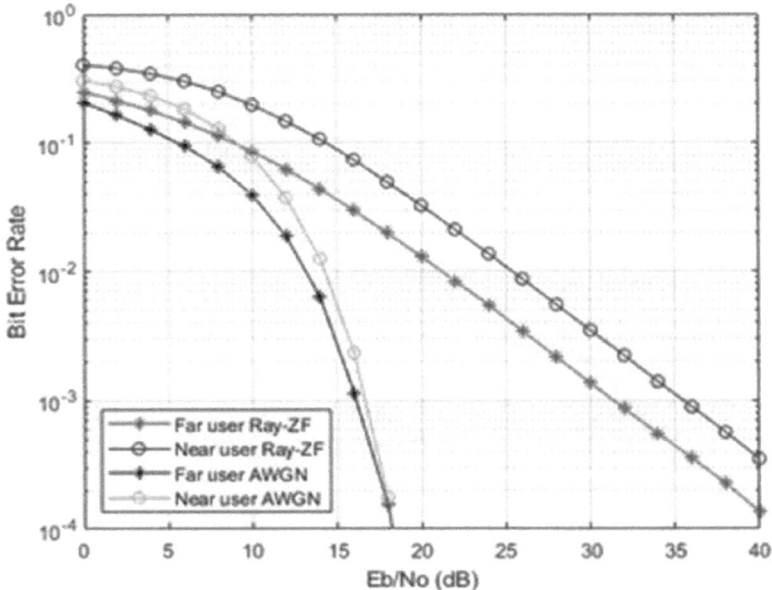

FIGURE 5.7   BER performance of PD-NOMA.

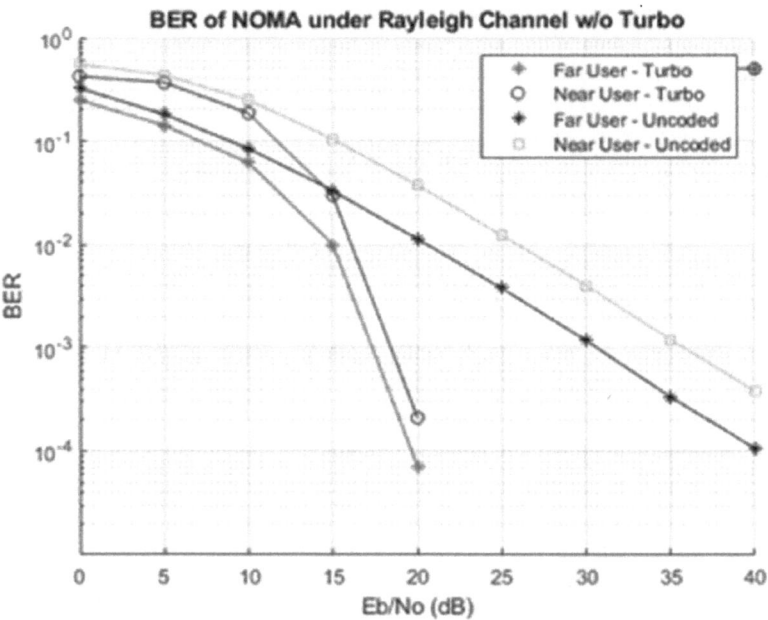

FIGURE 5.8   BER performance of PD-NOMA w/o turbo under a Rayleigh fading channel.

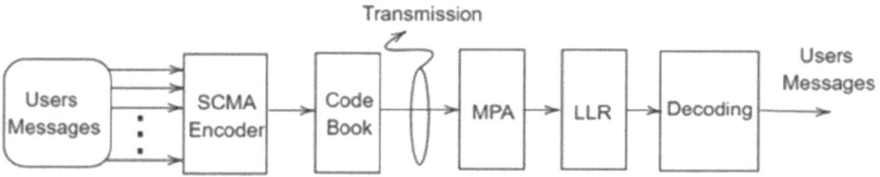

FIGURE 5.9 Code-domain NOMA schematic diagram.

algorithm (MPA) is a detection mechanism for multi-users used in SCMA decoding. The factor graph matrix includes two critical elements: (d f) which represents the total number of interfering users at a resource, and (d v) which represents the number of resources allotted to each user. With the number of users interfering with resources, the MPA complexity grows exponentially. The JK SCMA model in this research is 64 SCMA, which represents four resources shared by six users.

In SCMA, the user's signals are transmitted over the resources. every user has a codebook containing **M** by **K**-dimensional constellations. Each code-word x_{jm} contains $\mathbf{d}_v$ non-zero complex components. The "$\mathbf{log}_2(\mathbf{M})$" data bits are mapped in the **K**-dimensional code-word. The received signal at i^{th} user can be expressed as [21]:

$$y_i = diag\left(h_i\right)\sum_{j=1}^{J}\sqrt{P_j}x_j + n_i \tag{5.6}$$

where,

- $h_i = \left(h_{i1}, h_{i2}, ..., h_{iK}\right)$ is the channel gain vector,
- P_j is the power of each user signal,
- $x_j = x_{j1}, x_{j2}, ..., x_{jK}$ is the SCMA code-word of the jth user,
- n_i is additive white Gaussian noise (AWGN).

The SCMA structure in a factor graph matrix shown in Figure 5.10 is our proposed structure with $\mathbf{J} = 6, \mathbf{K}4$, and the corresponding matrix indicator **F** as follows:

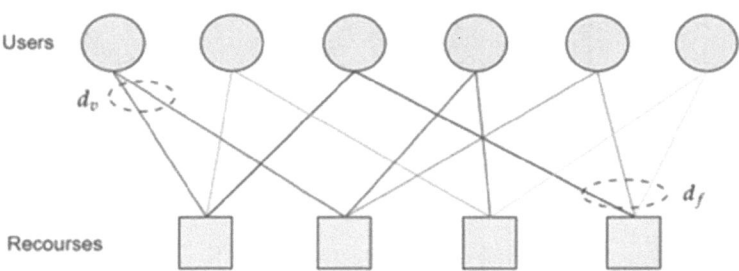

FIGURE 5.10 SCMA factor graph presentation with K = 4, J = 6, dv = 2 and df = 3.

$$\mathbf{F} = \begin{bmatrix} 1 & 1 & 1 & 0 & 0 & 0 \\ 1 & 0 & 0 & 1 & 1 & 0 \\ 0 & 1 & 0 & 1 & 0 & 1 \\ 0 & 0 & 1 & 0 & 1 & 1 \end{bmatrix} \qquad (5.7)$$

5.4.2.2 Message Passing Algorithm (MPA)

The code book is based on [22]. With the help of the sparsity of code words, the user detection for the system can be performed by MPA [23]. In MPA, resources and users' nodes exchange messages from each other to collect the users' data. A diagram for MPA is shown in Figure 5.11.

Below is an explanation of the steps for the SCMA Downlink system:

Step 1: Initialization
The prior probability of code-word x_j is uniform, hence:

$$g^0_{j\to k}\left(x_j\right) = P\left(x_j\right) = \frac{1}{M}, \forall j = 1, 2, \ldots, J, \forall K \in \Re\{j\} \qquad (5.8)$$

First, we obtain the f_n function:

$$f_n = \frac{-1}{\sigma^2}\left|y_k - \sum_{\{j \& x_{\{kj\}} \neq 0\}} h_{kj}x_{kj}\right|^2 \qquad (5.9)$$

Step 2: Iterative Message Exchange
Firstly, passing information from function nodes to Variable nodes:

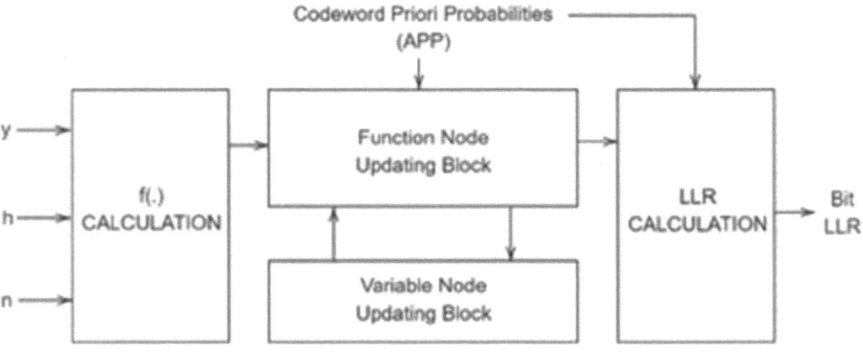

FIGURE 5.11   Diagram for message passing algorithm (MPA).

$$m_{k \to j}^{t}\left(x_{j}\right) = \sum_{\{x_{i} | i \in \mathbb{N}(k)/j\}} exp\{f_{n}\} \prod_{\{i \in \mathbb{N}(k)/j\}} g_{\{i \to k\}}^{\{t-1\}}\left(x\_i\right) \qquad (5.10)$$

Then, passing information from variable nodes to function nodes:

$$g_{\{j \to k\}}^{\{t\}}\left(x_{j}\right) = \frac{1}{M} \prod_{\{i \in \mathfrak{R}(j)/k\}} m_{\{i \to j\}}^{\{t-1\}}\left(x\_j\right) \qquad (5.11)$$

Then, normalization:

$$g_{\{j \to k\}}^{\{t\}}\left(x_{j}\right) = \frac{\prod_{\{i \in \mathfrak{R}(j)/k\}} m_{\{i \to j\}}^{\{t-1\}}\left(x_{j}\right)}{\sum_{x_{j}} \prod_{\{i \in \mathfrak{R}(j)/k\}} m_{\{i \to j\}}^{\{t-1\}}\left(x_{j}\right)} \qquad (5.12)$$

Step 3: LLR Calculation
A posteriori probability of the code-word x_{j} is defined as $Pr\left(x_{j}\right)$:

$$Pr\left(x_{j}\right) = \frac{1}{m} \prod_{\{k \in \mathfrak{R}(j)\}} m_{\{k \to j\}}^{\{T\}}\left(x_{j}\right) \qquad (5.13)$$

The log-likelihood ratios (LLRs):

$$LLR\left(b_{i}\right) = log \frac{\sum_{x_{j} \in \S | b_{i}=0} Pr\left(x_{j}\right)}{\sum_{x_{j} \in \S | b_{i}=1} Pr\left(x_{j}\right)} \qquad (5.14)$$

Finally, each of the user bits, b_{i} with $i \in \{1, 2, ..., \log_{2} M\}$ are estimated by:

$$\begin{cases} b_{i} = 1 & if\ LLR < 0 \\ b_{i} = 0 & otherwise \end{cases} \qquad (5.15)$$

5.4.2.3 Simulation Results

The bit error rate performance of the SCMA system shown in Figure 5.10 is implemented in MATLAB software. The SCMA system we are working with depends on MPA to extract the signals for the users. But on the other hand the complexity is high because of the exponential operations. The simulation result in Figure 5.12 shows the bit error rate for SCMA Downlink system under the Rayleigh fading channel for 6 users sharing 4 resources.

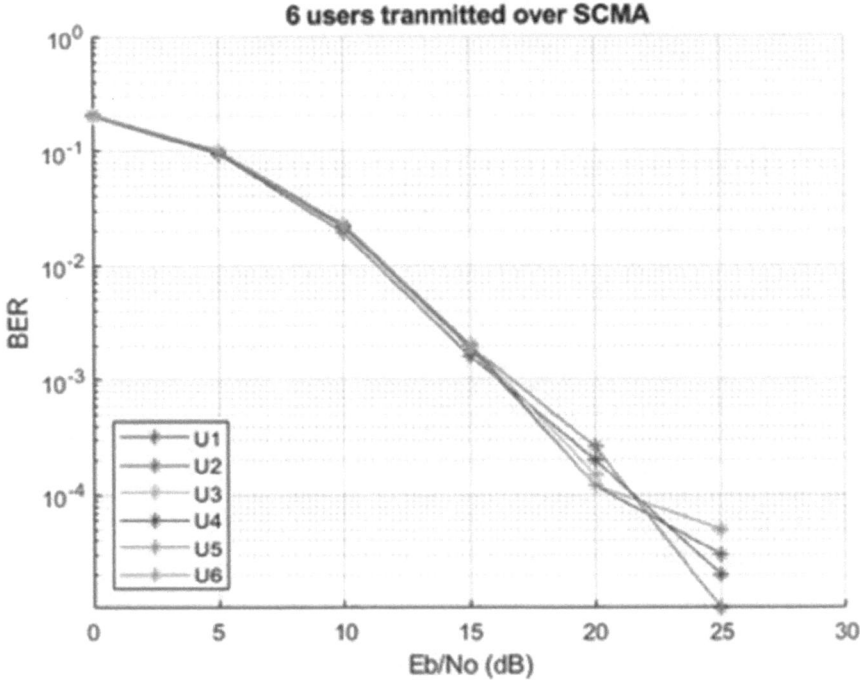

FIGURE 5.12   BER performance of an SCMA downlink.

5.4.3   Realistic Transmission Over the Rayleigh Fading Channel

In this section a realistic transmission over the Rayleigh fading channel is studied when using PD-NOMA.

5.4.3.1   System Models

Consider a single cell downlink network with one base station serving a set of users. The users are deployed randomly within the cell as shown in Figure 5.13. Then, the BS will compare two nearby of users' angles, the two users with angle differences of less than $\pi/12$ are considered as potential NOMA users. After that, the BS allocates to each of the pair a power according to their distance from the BS. In this scenario, we deployed 50 users randomly and we found the number of users configured as NOMA to be 24. Refer to Table 5.1 for a sample of the allocated power and distance for NOMA users. Furthermore, we retrieved all NOMA users' distances and powers allocated to them and apply that data on the downlink PD-NOMA system as shown in Figure 5.8. The simulation parameters used are shown in Table 5.2.

5.4.3.1.1   Transmitter

In the transmitter, we superimposed the transmitted signals using superposition modulation (SPM) as shown in Figure 5.4. The superimposed signal was as follows:

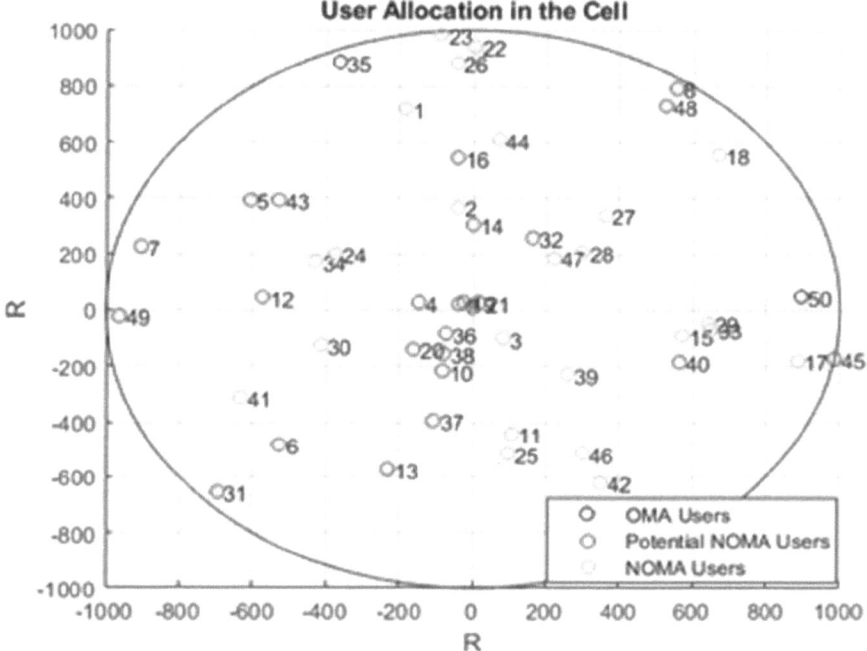

FIGURE 5.13 User allocation in cells around a base station.

TABLE 5.1
A Sample of Allocated Power and Distance for Users Configured as NOMA Users

Sig.	U	F/N	P	D	Sig.	U	F/N	P	D
1	1	Far	19.3	743	3	17	Far	15.3	904
1	2	Near	0.6	369	3	15	Near	4.6	578
2	39	Far	19.2	344	4	18	Far	18.6	870
2	3	Near	0.7	130	4	27	Near	1.3	496

Note: Sig.: Signal; U: Users; F/N: Far/Near; P: Power; and D: Distance.

$$x = r_1 s_{far} + r_2 s_{near} \tag{5.16}$$

Where $r_1 = \sqrt{P_1}$ and $r_2 = \sqrt{P_2}$, P_1 and P_2 are the powers allocated to each user subject to the condition that $r_1^2 + r_2^2 = 1$.

5.4.3.1.2 Receiver
In the receiver, zero forcing successive interference cancellation (ZF-SIC) is used. At the near user side, we decoded the far user signal first then re-modulated it to remove

TABLE 5.2
Simulation Parameters

Modulation Scheme	QPSK
Mapper Type	QPSK-SPM
Channel	Rayleigh Fading
Iterations	30
Bandwidth	20 MHz
Base Cell size	1000
Number of Bits	1e5
Number of Users in Cell	50 Users
Channel State Information (CSI)	Known
MUD Type	Zero Forcing

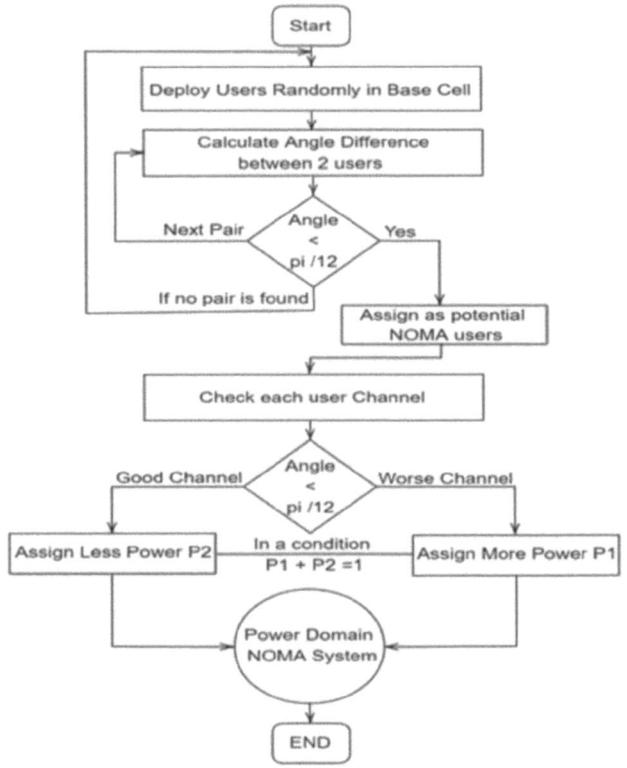

FIGURE 5.14   The flow chart of selecting the NOMA users from amongst all potential users shown in Figure 5.13.

its interference using the SIC method to decode the near user, denoted by s_{near} successively. At the far user side, we decoded the far user signal denoted by s_{far} directly without using SIC, assuming that the near user signal was due to the low power allocated to the user. It is assumed that the signal will be faded and will not reach the far user side. The receiver system is shown in Figure 5.8.

The flow chart of the decoding process is depicted in Figure 5.7.

The received signals at the two users, namely the far and near users can be defined as:

$$z_{far} = gx + n_{far} = g\left(r_1 s_{far} + r_2 s_{near}\right) + n_{far}$$

$$z_{near} = hx + n_{near} = h\left(r_1 s_{far} + r_2 s_{near}\right) + n_{near} \tag{5.17}$$

Where h and g represents the Rayleigh channel vector which is a zero mean complex circular Gaussian with co-variance matrix R_i for $i \in \{far, near\}$, and n_{near} and n_{far} are additive white Gaussian noise (AWGN).

Denoting ζ_{far} as the signal to interference plus noise ratio (SINR) to decode the far user message at the near user receiver signal s_{near} and ζ_{near} denotes the signal to noise ratio (SNR) to decode the near user message at its receiver s_{near}. So, we will have, at the near user receiver:

$$\zeta_{far} = \frac{\left|h^H r_1\right|^2}{\left|h^H r_2\right|^2 + \sigma^2_{near}} ; \zeta_{near} = \frac{\left|h^H r_2\right|^2}{\sigma^2_{near}} \tag{5.18}$$

Where h denotes the Rayleigh channel of the near user, and r_1, r_2 denote the power allocation to each user where r_1 is stronger than r_2 to make the decoding for the near user successful.

At the far user, the message for the far user is decoded directly because the signal of the near user will be faded as the signal is weak. We will have the SINR denoted as γ_{far} to decode the far user signal as:

$$\gamma_{far} = \frac{\left|g^H r_1\right|^2}{\left|g^H r_2\right|^2 + \sigma^2_{far}} \tag{5.19}$$

The achievable rates of decoding messages for far and near users are:

$$R_{far} = \frac{B}{U} log_2 \left(1 + \frac{P_{far} G_{far}}{G_{far} + \sigma^2}\right) \text{ and}$$

$$R_{near} = \frac{B}{U} log_2 \left(1 + \frac{P_{near} G_{near}}{\sigma^2} \right)$$

(5.20)

Where B denotes the bandwidth, U denotes the number of users and G denotes the channel gain.

5.4.3.2 Simulation Results

The bit error rate (BER) performance of near user s_{near} and far user s_{far} for the system shown in Figure 5.8 is calculated in different $\mathbf{Eb/N0}$ where the summation of power allocated to the two users must be equal to 1, which satisfies $r_1^2 + r_2^2 = 1$. The number of users considered as NOMA is 24 users from Figure 5.14. We used binary phase shift keying modulation (BPSK) to modulate users' signals. The simulation result in Figure 5.15 shows the BER performance for the PD-NOMA downlink system under the Rayleigh fading channel and shows that it gives a good performance.

We calculated the data rate for all NOMA users at each iteration as shown in Figure 5.16.

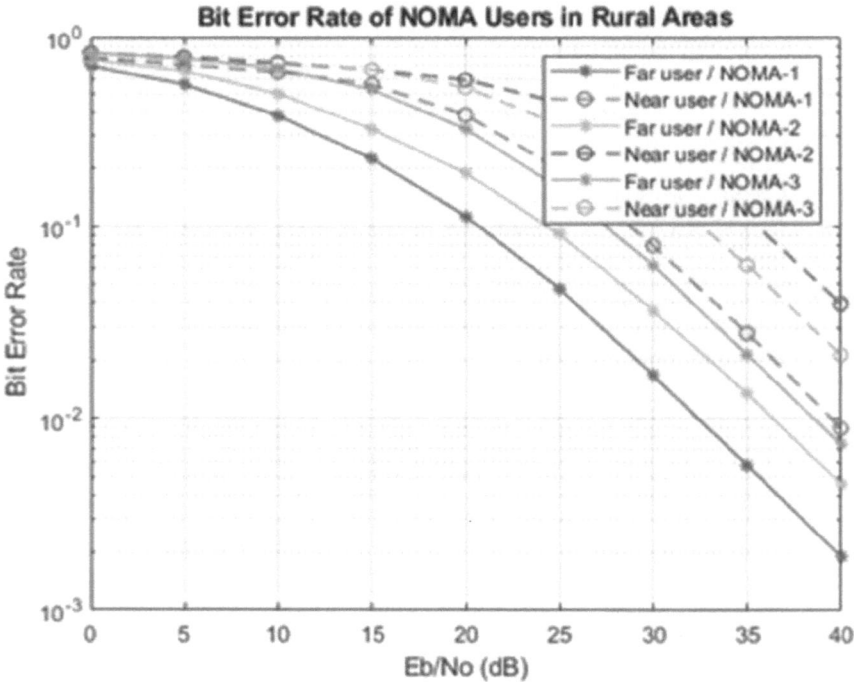

FIGURE 5.15 BER performance for users configured as NOMA users.

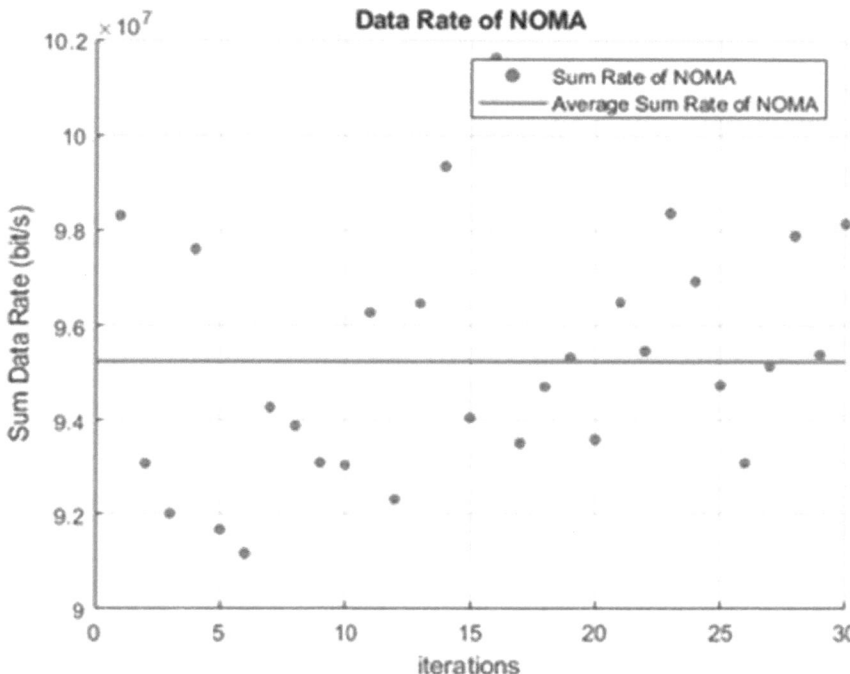

FIGURE 5.16 Data rate of NOMA users in rural areas.

5.5 CONCLUSION

Practical NOMA transmission is investigated using a variety of approaches. First, we constructed PD-NOMA using AWGN and Rayleigh channels, and then we used ZF to decode the data. Then we developed CD-NOMA, decoding using SCMA and extracting data from users with MPA. Finally, we implemented a realistic transmission scenario in which users were randomly assigned to cells and a downlink network with a single base station servicing a group of users was employed. The system demonstrates that not all possible NOMA users are regarded as NOMA users. Additionally, we created a downlink PD-NOMA for NOMA users and displayed the BER performance as well as the sum rate of NOMA users.

REFERENCES

1. Dai, L., Wang, B., Ding, Z., Wang, Z., Chen S., and Hanzo, L. "A survey of non-orthogonal multiple access for 5G," *IEEE Communications Surveys & Tutorials*, vol. 20, no. 3, pp. 2294–2323, third quarter. 2018.
2. Benjebbovu, A., Li, A., Saito, Y., Kishiyama, Y., Harada, A., and Nakamura, T. "System-level performance of downlink NOMA for future LTE enhancements," *2013 IEEE Globecom Workshops (GC Wkshps)*, Atlanta, GA, 2–13, pp. 66–70, 2013.

3. Saito, Y., Kishiyama, Y., Benjebbour, A., Nakamura, T. Li, A., and Higuchi, K. "Non-orthogonal multiple access (NOMA) for cellular future radio access," *2013 IEEE 77th Vehicular Technology Conference (VTC Spring)*, Dresden, pp. 1–5, 2013.
4. Sadia, H., Zeeshan, M., and Sheikh, S. A. "Performance analysis of downlink power domain NOMA under fading channels," *2018 ELEKTRO*, Mikulov, pp. 1–6, 2018.
5. Islam, S. M. R., Avazov, N., Dobre, O. A., and Kwak, K. "Power-domain non-o multiple access (NOMA) in 5G systems: Potentials and challenges," *IEEE Communications Surveys & Tutorials*, vol. 19, no. 2, pp. 721–742, Second quarter. 2017.
6. Wang, P., Xiao, J., and Ping, L. "Comparison of orthogonal and non-orthogonal approaches to future wireless cellular systems," *IEEE Vehicular Technology Magazine*, vol. 1, no. 3, pp. 4–11, Sept. 2006.
7. Wei, Z., Ng, D. W. K., and Yuan, J. "Power-efficient resource allocation for MC-NOMA with statistical channel state information," *2016 IEEE Global Communications Conference (GLOBECOM)*, Washington, DC, pp. 1–7, 2016.
8. Cai, Y. Qin, Z. Cui, F., Li, G. Y., and McCann, J. A. "Modulation and multiple access for 5G networks," *IEEE Communications Surveys & Tutorials*, vol. 20, no. 1, pp. 629–646, First quarter. 2018.
9. Choi, J. "NOMA: Principles and recent results," *2017 International Symposium on Wireless Communication Systems (ISWCS)*, Bologna, pp. 349–354, 2017.
10. Cai, W., Lv, G., and Jin, Y. "Half-ZF beamforming scheme for downlink two-user multiple input single output-based non-orthogonal multiple access systems," *IET Communications*, vol. 11, no. 10, pp. 1633–1640, 13 7, 2017.
11. Yang, J., and Huang, W. "Joint beamforming and power allocation design in non-orthogonal multiple access systems," *2016 International Computer Symposium (ICS)*, Chiayi, pp. 706–709, 2016.
12. Choi, J. "Minimum power multicast beamforming with superposition coding for multiresolution broadcast and application to NOMA systems," *IEEE Transactions on Communications*, vol. 63, no. 3, pp. 791–800, March 2015.
13. Choi, J. "On generalized downlink beamforming with NOMA," *Journal of Communications and Networks*, vol. 19, no. 4, pp. 319–328, August 2017.
14. Kimy, B., *et al.*, "Non-orthogonal multiple access in a downlink multiuser beamforming system," *MILCOM 2013–2013 IEEE Military Communications Conference*, San Diego, CA, pp. 1278–1283, 2013.
15. Ali, S., Hossain, E., and Kim, D. I. "Non-orthogonal multiple access (NOMA) for downlink multiuser MIMO systems: User clustering, beamforming, and power allocation," *IEEE Access*, vol. 5, pp. 565–577, 2017.
16. Anwar, A., Boon-Chong, S., Hasan, M., and Li, X. J. (2019). A survey on application of non-orthogonal multiple access to different wireless networks," *Electronics*. 8, p. 1355. 10.3390/electronics 8111355.
17. Cover, T. "Broadcast channels," *IEEE Transactions on Information Theory*, vol. 18, no. 1, pp. 2–14, January 1972.
18. Cho, Y. S., Kim, J., Yang, W. Y., and Kang, C. G. " MIMO-OFDM wireless communications with MATLAB," in *IEEE Press*, Wiley, UK, pp. 9–16, 2011.
19. Ohwatari, Y., Miki, N., Asai, T., Abe, T., and Taoka, H. "Performance of advanced receiver employing interference rejection combining to suppress inter-cell interference in LTE-advanced downlink," *2011 IEEE Vehicular Technology Conference (VTC Fall)*, San Francisco, CA, pp. 1–7, 2011.
20. Nikopour, H., and Baligh, H. "Sparse code multiple access," *2013 IEEE 24th Annual International Symposium on Personal, Indoor, and Mobile Radio Communications (PIMRC)*, London, pp. 332–336, 2013.

21. Lai, K. Lei, J. Wen, L. Chen, G. Li, W., and Xiao, P. "Secure transmission with randomized constellation rotation for downlink sparse code multiple access system," *IEEE Access*, vol. 6, pp. 5049–5063, 2018.
22. Zhang, S., *et al.*, "A capacity-based codebook design method for sparse code multiple access systems," *2016 8th International Conference on Wireless Communications & Signal Processing (WCSP)*, Yangzhou, pp. 1–5, 2016.
23. Nikopour, H., *et al.*, "SCMA for downlink multiple access of 5G wireless networks," *2014 IEEE Global Communications Conference*, Austin, TX, pp. 3940–3945, 2014.

6 Comparisons of UTD-PO and FKE Models for Path Loss Prediction over an Irregular Terrain

Yashu Shanker and D. K. Lobiyal

CONTENTS

6.1 INTRODUCTION

In last few decades, path loss prediction of mobile radio wave propagation over an irregular terrain has been one of the major challenges for researchers [1]. As the terrains are inherently irregular and diverse in nature, the received field varies arbitrarily as a receiver moves across them [2–6]. Therefore, path loss prediction is very difficult. The researcher working in this area must take into account the major aspects of obstacles such as their height, shape, position and measurement terrain data [7–8]. Based on these aspects, several approaches have been developed. This includes ray tracing, the diffraction mechanism, and Fresnel theory that are applied in deterministic modeling approaches. However, empirical modeling based on terrain measurement data is preferred to precisely predicting path loss over terrains. Later on, semi deterministic models are also proposed. Both the empirical and deterministic approaches are used to develop these models. The series of irregular terrain profiles [9–12] are approximated as knife-edge obstacles. In this, it is assumed that diffraction takes place only over the rooftop of the knife edge obstacles and it is explained by the Huygens Fresnel principle. Fresnel zone geometry and Fresnel-Kirchhoff knife edge diffraction parameters explain the diffraction loss in the Fresnel-Kirchhoff knife edge diffraction FKE model [13].

DOI: 10.1201/9781003368311-6

In the literature, a theoretical model for the prediction of path loss for radio propagation due to multiple diffractions across a series of obstacles of uniform height and spacing was proposed by Bertoni *et al.* [14]. This proposed approach is used only when the height of the transmitter is above the height of the obstacle, and the series of obstacles is of uniform height and spacing. Therefore, this model is not applicable to the urban microcellular scenario. Later on, Saunders *et al.* [15] proposed an attenuation function as an explicit solution for multiple diffractions over a series of a large number of obstacles. Also, it extended the solution for arbitrary height and spacing of the series of obstacles using a numerical method [16].

In [17], the authors studied the impact of obstacle height variation when undergoing multiple diffractions to predict path loss. Then Tzaras *et al.* [18] proposed an improved solution, namely, the uniform theory of diffraction (UTD) with slope diffraction coefficient of higher order for a series of obstacles approximated as a knife edge for arbitrary height and spacing. Later Koutitas *et al.* [19] improved the sloped UTD solution by proposing it for multi-shaped multiple obstacles but it increased the mathematical and computational complexity of the solution. Rodriguez *et al.* [20–21] proposed a new solution that reduced the mathematical complexity by removing the slope term from the uniform theory of diffraction-physical optics UTD-PO solution. But this solution is only applicable to a series of obstacles, namely, knife-edge of uniform height and spacing. In this paper, we compared UTD-PO and FKE models for path loss prediction due to over-rooftop multiple diffractions over an irregular terrain scenario for mobile radio propagation [22–30]. The results obtained from the models are validated with the measurement data available in the literature.

A representation of the work presented in this paper is given below. Section II briefly explains the propagation environment for this technique. Section III explains the UTD-PO and FKE models for the computation of path loss over the irregular terrain scenario. In Section IV, both of the models are validated for irregular terrain scenarios, and the results obtained are compared with the available measurement data

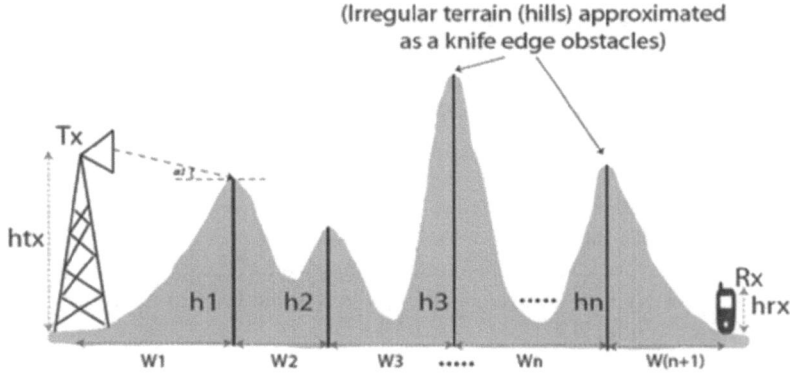

FIGURE 6.1   A symbolic representation of a propagation scenario over an irregular terrain.

for such a terrain environment. Finally in Section V the work presented in the paper is concluded.

6.1.1 PROPAGATION ENVIRONMENT

Figure 6.1 shows the schematic representation of a transmitter T_x of height h_{tx} which is propagating spherical waves to a receiving point or moving mobile unit R_x of height h_{rx} over an irregular terrain. There is a series of obstacles of uneven height (namely, $h_1, h_2, h_3, \ldots, h_n$) and spacing (namely, $w_1, w_2, w_3, \ldots, w_n, w_{(n+1)}$) between them. This series of obstacles are approximated as knife edge obstacles in which the only contribution to path loss is due to over-rooftop knife edge diffraction. In this, a spherical wave impinges on the rooftop of a knife edge obstacle at some angle of incidence when propagating from transmitter T_x. In Figure 6.1, an angle α_1 represents the angle of incidence for obstacle 1 for a wave propagating from the transmitter. Similarly different obstacles of uneven height and spacing have their different angles of incidence which are used for the computation of path loss due to multiple over-rooftop diffraction.

6.2 PROPOSED ANALYSIS

The proposed comparative study is done for path loss analysis for radio wave propagation over the irregular terrain scenario as shown in Figure 6.1. The path loss is predicted for the case when the receiver R_x or mobile unit is moving away from the transmitter T_x over a terrain having obstacles or hills of uneven height and spacing. For the prediction of path loss using the uniform theory of diffraction-physical optics UTD-PO and Fresnel-Kirchhoff knife edge diffraction theory FKE is applied.

First, we calculate the path loss over an irregular terrain using a UTD-PO approach. It is a high-frequency electromagnetic field approximation approach which is used to determine the effect of radio propagation mechanism, for example, diffraction, interference, polarization, and so forth, for which other ray tracing approaches are not valid. UTD-PO is used to resolve issues related to the scattering of radio waves in the shadow region of the obstacles. This field is computed uniformly in the shadow region without any discontinuities in the prediction of the field. A ray diffraction model is used to determine the diffraction coefficient of a knife edge for each diffracting wave. These diffraction coefficients determine the received field strength and the phase factor of the propagating wave after diffraction from the roof top of the knife edge obstacle. The total solution is obtained by adding these received fields with their corresponding incident and reflected fields.

By applying the above approaches, we calculate the total received field at the receiver R_x a wave arrived by passing through a series of obstacles or a hill of n-dimensions (face). This series of obstacles is approximated as knife edge obstacles of arbitrary height and spacing. When the 0th-face and the nth-face of an obstacle or a hill are equal, a single half-screen or a knife edge is used to depict the obstacle as shown in Figures 6.2, 6.3, 6.4, 6.5 6.6 and 6.7.

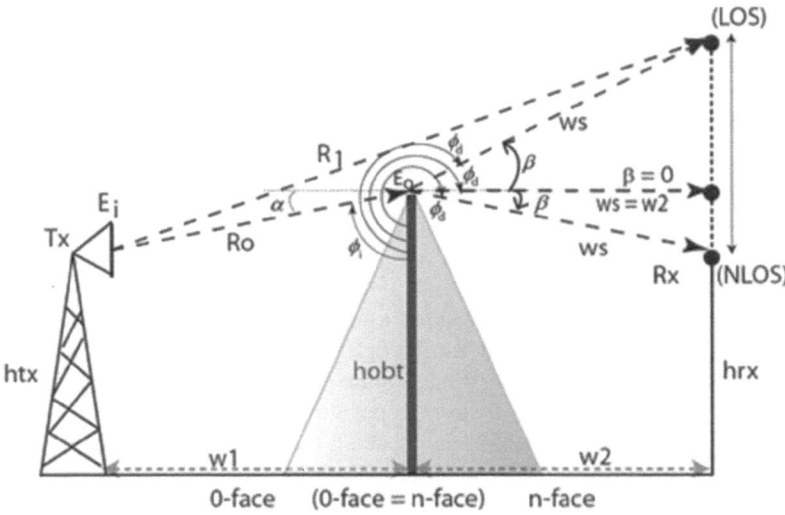

FIGURE 6.2   The height of the transmitter is below the height of the obstacle, and the receiver moves from NLOS to LOS.

For the calculation of the received field, we considered a spherical radio wave that impinges on the knife edge obstacle such that the incident field E_o is given by

$$E_o = \frac{E_i}{R_o} . \exp\left(-jkR_o\right)$$

(6.1)

Where E_i is the field transmitted from the transmitter T_x, and its value is unity.

R_o is the radial distance between the transmitter T_x and the knife edge obstacle as shown in Figures 6.2, 6.3 and 6.4.

Categorization of an irregular terrain scenario based on relative knife edge obstacle height $h_{obt,}$ with respect to the height of the transmitting point h_{tx} and the receiving point h_{rx}:

Case 1: When the transmitter T_x of height h_{tx} is below the height of obstacle $h_{obt,}$ and the receiving point R_x of height h_{rx} is moving vertically from NLOS (no line-of-sight) to LOS (line-of-sight) as shown in Figure 6.2.

The received field E_r at the receiving point when receiver R_x is below the NLOS is given as

$$E_r = E_0\left[\sqrt{\frac{R_0}{w_s\left(R_0 + w_s\right)}} . D\left(\phi_i, \phi_d, L\right) . \exp\left(-jkw_s\right)\right]$$

(6.2)

$$D\left(\phi_i, \phi_d, L\right) = D\left(\phi_i = \frac{\pi}{2} - \alpha, \phi_d = \frac{3\pi}{2} + \beta, L = \frac{R_0 . w_s}{R_0 + w_s}\right)$$

(6.3)

The received field E_r at the receiving point when the receiver R_x is moved above the LOS is given as

$$E_r = E_0 \left[\frac{R_0}{R_1}.\exp\left(-jk\left(R_1 - R_0\right)\right) + \sqrt{\frac{R_0}{w_s\left(R_0 + w_s\right)}}.D\left(\phi_i,\phi_d,L\right).\exp\left(-jkw_s\right) \right] \quad (6.4)$$

$$D\left(\phi_i,\phi_d,L\right) = D\left(\phi_i = \frac{\pi}{2} - \alpha, \phi_d = \frac{3\pi}{2} - \beta, L = \frac{R_0.w_s}{R_0 + w_s} \right) \quad (6.5)$$

Where,
$$R_o = \sqrt{\left(h_{tx} - h_{obt}\right)^2 + \left(w_1\right)^2} \quad (6.6)$$

$$R_1 = \sqrt{\left(h_{tx} - h_{rx}\right)^2 + \left(w_1 + w_2\right)^2} \quad (6.7)$$

$$w_s = \sqrt{\left(h_{obt} - h_{rx}\right)^2 + \left(w_2\right)^2} \quad (6.8)$$

$$k = \frac{2\pi}{\lambda} \quad (6.9)$$

Where:
k represents the wave number,
$D\left(\phi_i,\phi_d,L\right)$ represents the knife edge diffraction coefficient [18],
ϕ_i represents the incident angle from the 0th face of the knife edge obstacle,
ϕ_d represents the diffracted angle from the 0th face of the knife edge obstacle,
L represents the distance parameter,
R_1 represents the radial distance between the transmitter T_x and the receiver T_x,
w_1 represents the geometric distance between the transmitter T_x and the knife edge obstacle,
w_2 represents the geometric distance between the knife edge obstacle and the receiver T_x,
w_s represents the radial distance between the knife edge obstacle and the receiver T_x.

Case 2: When the height h_{tx} of the transmitter T_x is equal to the height of obstacle h_{obt} and the receiving point R_x of height h_{rx} is moving vertically from NLOS to LOS as shown in Figure 6.3.
The received field E_r at the receiving point when receiver R_x is below the NLOS and is given as

$$E_r = E_0 \left[\sqrt{\frac{R_0}{w_s\left(R_0 + w_s\right)}}.D\left(\phi_i,\phi_d,L\right).\exp\left(-jkw_s\right) \right] \quad (6.10)$$

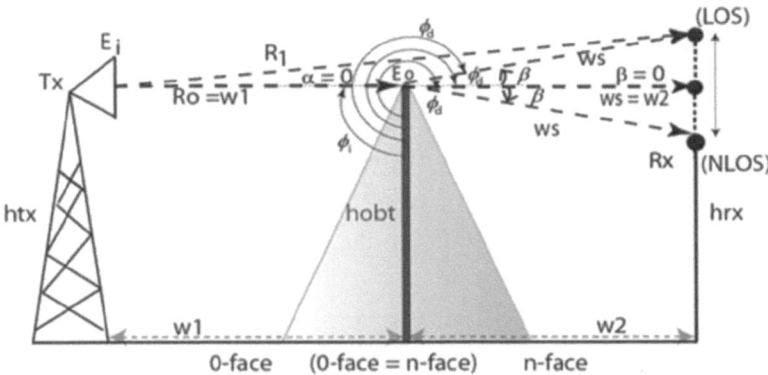

FIGURE 6.3 The height of the transmitter is equal to the height of the obstacle, and the receiver moves from NLOS to LOS.

$$D\left(\phi_i,\phi_d,L\right) = D\left(\phi_i = \frac{\pi}{2},\phi_d = \frac{3\pi}{2}+\beta, L = \frac{R_0.w_s}{R_0+w_s}\right) \tag{6.11}$$

The received field E_r at the receiving point when the receiver R_x is moved above the LOS and is given as

$$E_r = E_0 \left[\begin{array}{c} \dfrac{R_0}{R_1}.\exp\left(-jk\left(R_1-R_0\right)\right)+ \\[2ex] \sqrt{\dfrac{R_0}{w_s\left(R_0+w_s\right)}}.D\left(\phi_i,\phi_d,L\right).\exp\left(-jkw_s\right) \end{array} \right] \tag{6.12}$$

$$D\left(\phi_i,\phi_d,L\right) = D\left(\phi_i = \frac{\pi}{2},\phi_d = \frac{3\pi}{2}-\beta, L = \frac{R_0.w_s}{R_0+w_s}\right) \tag{6.13}$$

All the parameters are defined in Case 1.

Case 3: When the transmitter T_x of height h_{tx} is above the height of obstacle h_{obt} and the receiving point R_x of height h_{rx} is moving vertically from NLOS to LOS as shown in Figure 6.4.

The received field E_r at the receiving point when receiver R_x is below the NLOS is given as

$$E_r = E_0 \left[\sqrt{\frac{R_0}{w_s\left(R_0+w_s\right)}}.D\left(\phi_i,\phi_d,L\right).\exp\left(-jkw_s\right) \right] \tag{6.14}$$

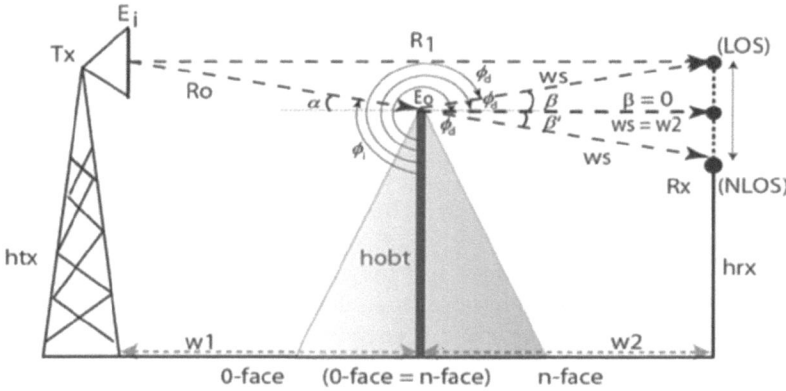

FIGURE 6.4 The height of the transmitter is above the height of the obstacle and the receiver moves from NLOS to LOS.

$$D\left(\phi_i,\phi_d,L\right)= D\left(\phi_i = \frac{\pi}{2}+\alpha, \phi_d = \frac{3\pi}{2}+\beta, L = \frac{R_0.w_s}{R_0 + w_s}\right) \qquad (6.15)$$

The received field E_r at the receiving point when the receiver R_x is moved above LOS is given as

$$E_r = E_0\left[\begin{array}{c} \dfrac{R_0}{R_1}.\exp\left(-jk\left(R_1 - R_0\right)\right)+ \\ \sqrt{\dfrac{R_0}{w_s\left(R_0 + w_s\right)}}.D\left(\phi_i,\phi_d,L\right).\exp\left(-jkw_s\right) \end{array}\right] \qquad (6.16)$$

$$D\left(\phi_i,\phi_d,L\right)= D\left(\phi_i = \frac{\pi}{2}+\alpha, \phi_d = \frac{3\pi}{2}-\beta, L = \frac{R_0.w_s}{R_0 + w_s}\right) \qquad (6.17)$$

All the parameters are defined in Case 1.

Consideration of the three cases

The above cases consider all of the possible scenarios for the prediction of the received field over a series of obstacles (namely, irregular terrain) using the UTD-PO approach. Also, during the prediction of the field over multiple obstacles, the received field at any intermediate points is considered as a point source or virtual transmitting point to predict the field further. In this way, we have considered all of the possible paths between the transmitting and the receiving point to compute the received fields when the receiver if moved vertically from NLOS to LOS.

Now, the path loss for using the UTD-PO approach to knife edge obstacles is given as

$$L(dB) = -20.\log_{10} \left| \frac{E_r}{E_o'} \right| \qquad (6.18)$$

E_o' is the free space electric field with no obstacles present between the transmitting and the receiving points.

Now, we calculate the path loss over irregular terrain using the FKE approach. Prediction of path loss for radio propagation due to diffraction of radio waves over irregular terrain is difficult because it is complex in nature. Therefore, the irregular terrain is considered as a knife edge or single screen obstacles having equal 0th-face and n^{th}-face. This way we reduce the structural complexity of the irregular terrain scenario to study the proposed approach. In this approach, we consider a knife edge obstacle of relative effective height h_{oeff} with an infinite width such that no propagation takes place through the sides of the knife edge obstacles. Propagation only takes place through the rooftop of the knife edge obstacles. This obstacle is placed at geometric distance w_1 and radial distance d_1 from the transmitter T_x of height h_{tx} and at geometric distance w_2 and radial distance d_2 from the receiver R_x of height h_{rx} as shown in Figures 6.5, 6.6, 6.7 and 6.8.

When transmitter T_x propagates radio waves to the receiver R_x via the rooftop of the knife edge obstacles, waves get diffracted from the rooftop of the knife edge obstacles. These diffracted radio waves take longer paths than the direct ray path (namely, the line-of-sight path). In this situation we have to determine the excess path length ($\varnothing$) between the diffracted ray and the direct ray path, such that $h_{oeff} \ll d_1$, d_2 and $h_{oeff} \gg \lambda$ where λ is the wavelength.

$$\Delta = \frac{h_{oeff}^2}{2} \cdot \left(\frac{1}{d_1} + \frac{1}{d_2} \right) \qquad (6.19)$$

Now its corresponding phase difference is given as

$$\varphi = \frac{2\pi}{\lambda} \cdot (\Delta) \qquad (6.20)$$

From Equations (6.18) and (6.19), we get

$$\varphi = \frac{2\pi}{\lambda} \cdot \left(\frac{h_{oeff}^2}{2} \cdot \left(\frac{1}{d_1} + \frac{1}{d_2} \right) \right) \qquad (6.21)$$

$$\varphi = \pi \cdot \left(\frac{h_{oeff}^2}{\lambda} \cdot \left(\frac{1}{d_1} + \frac{1}{d_2} \right) \right) \qquad (6.22)$$

$$\varphi = \frac{\pi}{2} \cdot \left(\frac{2h_{oeff}^2}{\lambda} \cdot \left(\frac{1}{d_1} + \frac{1}{d_2} \right) \right)$$

(6.23)

Equations (6.22) and (6.23), show that the direct ray and the diffracted ray path are π radians out of phase. This means that there is a $\frac{1}{2}$ cycle difference in the path of both rays at any point in time.

$$\varphi = \frac{\pi}{2} \cdot v^2$$

(6.24)

$$v = h_{oeff} \cdot \sqrt{\frac{2}{\lambda} \cdot \left(\frac{1}{d_1} + \frac{1}{d_2} \right)}$$

(6.25)

Equation (6.23) is simplified in Equation (6.24) by using dimensionless Fresnel-Kirchhoff diffraction parameter v given in Equation (6.25). Equation (6.24) shows that the phase difference between both rays is a function of effective height and effective distance of the obstacle with respect to the position of the T_x and R_x.

When the receiver R_x is in the shadowed region, namely, behind the obstacle where no line-of-sight exists, the received field at R_x is the vector sum of all the fields from the rooftop of the knife edge obstacle. For this, the v-parameter is used to determine the received field at the receiver R_x.

Categorization of an irregular terrain scenario based on effective knife edge obstacle height h_{oeff}, relative height h_{tx} of the transmitter, and height h_{rx} of the receiver.

Case 1: The height h_{tx} of the transmitter T_x and height h_{rx} of the receiver R_x are below the effective height h_{oeff} of an obstacle and no line-of-sight exists between the T_x and the R_x as shown in Figure 6.5.

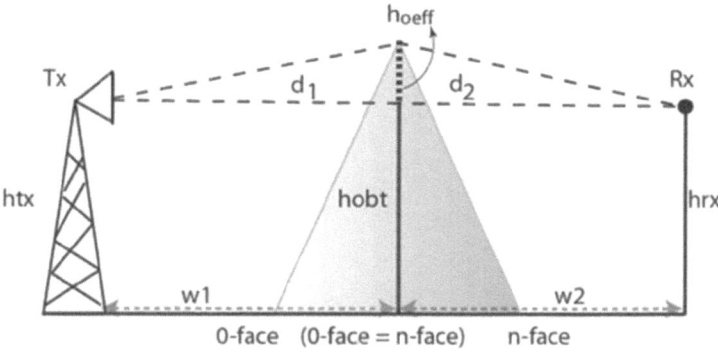

FIGURE 6.5 The height of the transmitter and the receiver are below the effective height of the knife edge obstacle.

The dimensionless Fresnel-Kirchhoff knife edge diffraction parameter v is given as

$$v = h_{oeff} \cdot \sqrt{\frac{2}{\lambda}\left(\frac{1}{d_1} + \frac{1}{d_2}\right)} \qquad (6.26)$$

$$d_1 = \sqrt{\left(h_{tx} - h_{obt}\right)^2 + \left(w_1\right)^2} \qquad (6.27)$$

$$d_2 = \sqrt{\left(h_{obt} - h_{rx}\right)^2 + \left(w_2\right)^2} \qquad (6.28)$$

Case 2: The relative height h_{tx} of the transmitter T_x and height h_{rx} of the receiver R_x are equal and LOS exists between the T_x and the R_x. Therefore, the effective height h_{oeff} of the obstacle is zero as shown in Figure 6.6.
Dimensionless Fresnel-Kirchhoff knife edge diffraction parameter v is given as

$$v = \left(h_{oeff} = 0\right) \cdot \sqrt{\frac{2}{\lambda}\left(\frac{1}{d_1} + \frac{1}{d_2}\right)} = 0 \qquad (6.29)$$

All the parameters are defined in Case 1.
Case 3: The height h_{tx} of the transmitter T_x and the height h_{rx} of the receiver R_x are above the effective height h_{oeff} of an obstacle and the LOS exists between the T_x and the R_x as shown in Figure 6.7.
Dimensionless Fresnel-Kirchhoff knife edge diffraction parameter v is given as

$$v = -h_{oeff} \cdot \sqrt{\frac{2}{\lambda}\left(\frac{1}{d_1} + \frac{1}{d_2}\right)} \qquad (6.30)$$

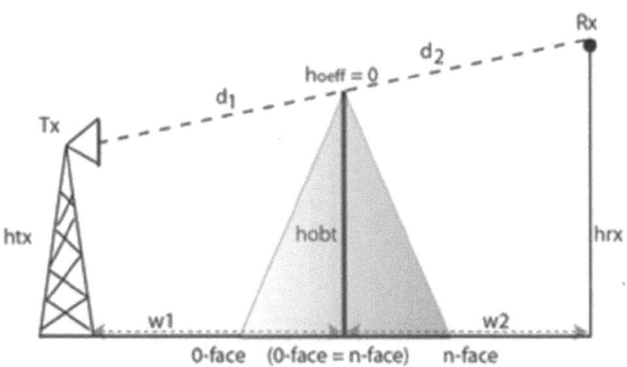

FIGURE 6.6 The height of the transmitter and height of the receiver are adjusted such that the relative effective height of the knife edge obstacle is zero.

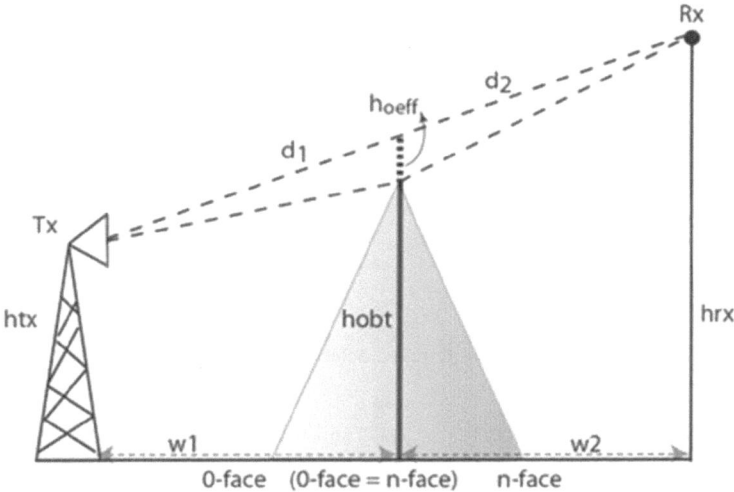

Rx

htx

Tx

d1

hoeff

d2

hobt

hrx

w1   w2

0-face   (0-face = n-face)   n-face

FIGURE 6.7   The height of the transmitter and height of the receiver are above the effective height of the knife edge of the obstacle.

All the parameters are defined in Case 1.

Consideration of the three cases

The above cases of the FKE approach considered all the possibilities for computing Fresnel-Kirchhoff knife edge diffraction parameter '*v*' over an irregular terrain scenario from NLOS to LOS. This value of *v*-parameter is used to predict normalized electric field strength E_d with respect to free space electric field E_o, namely, when no obstacle is present between the transmitting and the receiving point as given in Equation (6.31).

$$\frac{E_d}{E_o} = F(v) = \frac{(1+j)}{2} \int_v^\infty \exp((j\pi t^2)/2).dt \qquad (6.31)$$

where F(*v*) is the complex Fresnel integral function of the Fresnel-Kirchhoff diffraction parameter *v*.

Now, the diffraction loss due to propagation over knife edge obstacles is given as

$$L(dB) = -20.\log_{10}|F(v)| \qquad (6.32)$$

Figure 6.8 shows the equivalent representation of knife-edge diffraction geometry which is used to compute the effective height of the knife edge obstacle h_{oeff} and the radial distance d_1 between the knife edge obstacle and the transmitter T_x, the radial distance d_2 between the knife edge obstacle and the receiver R_x as given in Equations (6.33) to (6.39).

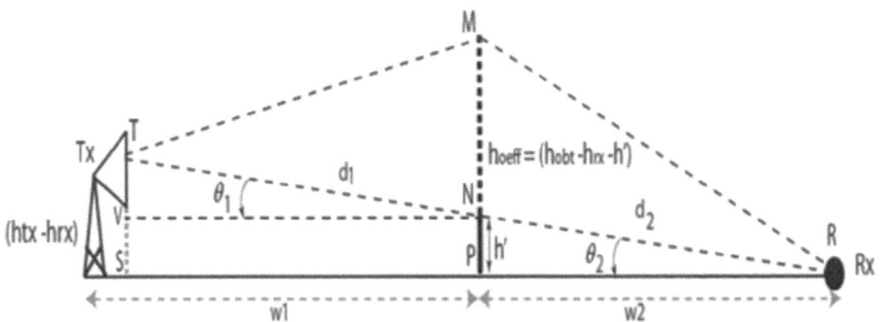

FIGURE 6.8 The equivalent geometric representation of the knife-edge diffraction model.

To calculate the effective height h_{oeff} of the knife edge obstacle, we first find the value of h'.

$$\tan(\theta_2) = \frac{h_{tx} - h_{rx}}{w_1 + w_2} \tag{6.33}$$

$$\tan(\theta_2) = \frac{h'}{w_2} \tag{6.34}$$

On comparing Equation (6.33) and (6.34), we get

$$h' = \left(\frac{w_2 (h_{tx} - h_{rx})}{w_1 + w_2} \right) \tag{6.35}$$

Now the radial distances d_1 and d_2 are calculated using Figure 6.8 and Equation (6.35) here, we get

$$d_2 = \sqrt{(h')^2 + (w_2)^2} \tag{6.36}$$

$$d_1 = \sqrt{(h_{tx} - h_{rx} - h')^2 + (w_1)^2} \tag{6.37}$$

Now, effective height of the knife edge obstacle is calculated using Equation (6.35)

$$h_{oeff} = (h_{obt} - h_{rx} - h') \tag{6.38}$$

$$h_{oeff} = \left(h_{obt} - h_{rx} - \left(\frac{w_2 (h_{tx} - h_{rx})}{w_1 + w_2} \right) \right) \tag{6.39}$$

In Giovaneli [11], a Fresnel-Kirchhoff knife edge diffraction approach is used to compute path loss over multiple obstacles. Absolute path loss is defined in this approach as the sum of the path losses determined from each individual obstacle with regard to Tx and Rx, without considering the impact of other obstacles.

6.3 RESULTS AND DISCUSSION

To validate UTD-PO and FKE approaches, four different terrain scenarios were chosen from the literature. MATLAB software is used to run all of the simulations. In Figures 6.9, 6.10, 6.11 and 6.12 the results obtained for the UTD-PO and the FKE approaches are compared with the measurement data observed at 25 GHz frequency vertically polarized [22]. For each of the following terrain scenarios, a simulation was run to estimate path loss for both approaches when the receiver moved vertically from NLOS (shadowed region) to LOS (illuminated region).

Figure 6.9 shows the prediction of path loss over a single knife edge obstacle where transmitter T_x of height h_{tx} is 58.33λ above the obstacle height h_{obt}, namely, 42.83λ and placed 105.25λ away from the obstacle. The receiver R_x has been placed 120.25λ away from the obstacle in the shadowed region, in other words, where no line-of-sight communication takes place. Propagation path loss is predicted when the receiver moves from *NLOS* to *LOS* vertically. The obtained path loss results for the UTD-PO and the FKE approaches show the same results when compared with the measurement data available for the single knife edge obstacle. Table 6.1 shows that the estimated path loss results obtained for the UTD-PO and the FKE approaches had mean errors of 0.6443 dB and 0.6445 dB, respectively. When compared to the mean error result predicted for the FKE approach, the predicted result for the UTD-PO

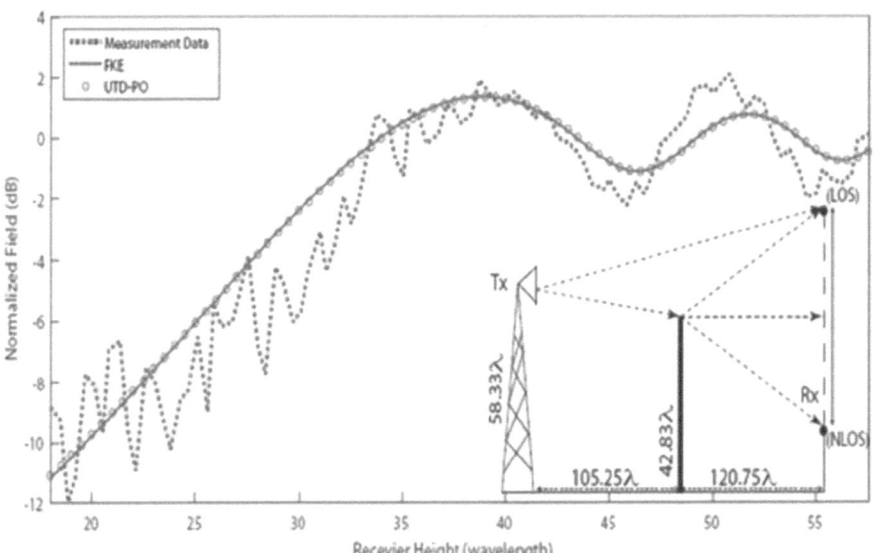

FIGURE 6.9 A comparison of results obtained for the path loss of a single knife edge obstacle for the UTD-PO and the FKE approach with the available measurement data.

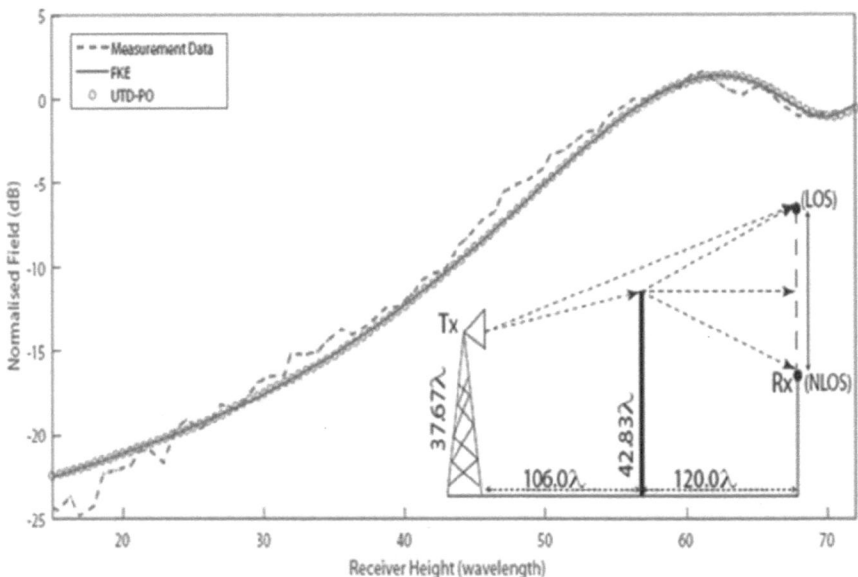

FIGURE 6.10 A comparison of the path loss obtained for a single knife edge obstacle using the UTD-PO and the FKE approaches with the available measurement data.

approach indicates a marginal improvement of 0.0002 dB. Also, data analysis for a single knife edge obstacle when transmitter T_x is above the obstacle shows that the UTD-PO and the FKE approaches give the same results.

Figure 6.10 shows the prediction of path loss over a single knife edge obstacle where transmitter T_x is of height h_{tx} 37.67 λ below the obstacle height h_{obt}, which is 42.83 λ and placed 106.9 λ away from the obstacle. The receiver R_x is placed 120.0 λ away from the obstacle in the shadowed region, namely, *NLOS*. Propagation path loss is predicted when the receiver moves from *NLOS* to *LOS* vertically. The path loss results obtained for the UTD-PO and the FKE approaches show the same results when compared with the measurement data available for the single knife edge obstacle. Table 6.1 shows that the estimated path loss results obtained for the UTD-PO and the FKE approaches had mean errors of 0.2647 dB and 0.2648 db, respectively. When compared to the mean error result predicted for the FKE approach, the predicted result for the UTD-PO approach indicates a marginal improvement of 0.0001 dB. Also, data analysis for single knife edge obstacle when transmitter T_x is below the obstacle shows that the UTD-PO and the FKE approaches give the same results.

Figure 6.11 shows the prediction of path loss over two knife edge obstacles where transmitter T_x of height h_{tx} 39.17 λ is below the first obstacle of height h_{obt1} of 42.83 λ and it is placed 96.08 λ away from the first obstacle. The second obstacle of height h_{obt2} of 42.83 λ is placed 16.91 λ away from the first obstacle. The receiver R_x is placed 96.08 λ away from the second obstacle in the shadowed region. Propagation path loss is predicted when the receiver moves from *NLOS* to *LOS* vertically. The path loss

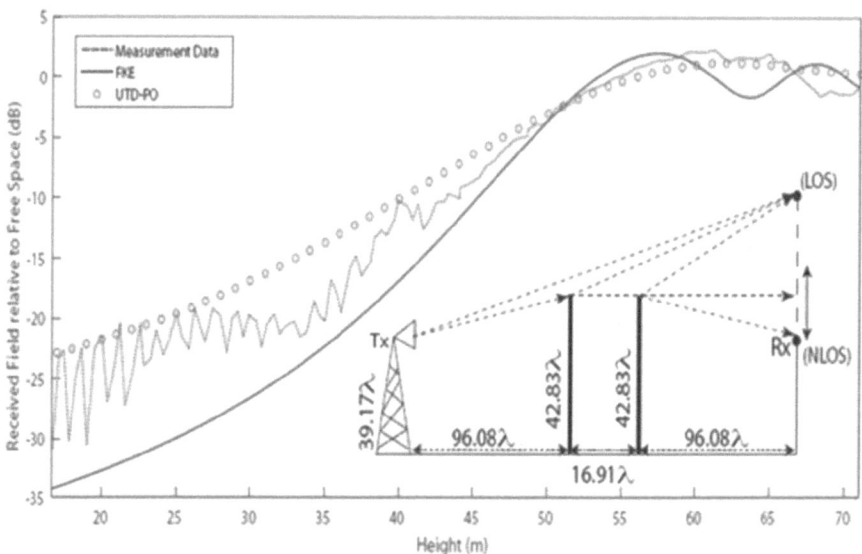

FIGURE 6.11 A comparison of the path loss obtained for two knife edge obstacles using the UTD-PO and the FKE approaches with the available measurement data.

results obtained for the UTD-PO and the FKE approaches show the same results when compared with the measurement data available for the two-knife edge obstacle. Table 6.1 shows that the estimated path loss results obtained for the UTD-PO and the FKE approaches had mean errors of 1.2192 dB and 2.7065 dB, respectively. When compared to the mean error result predicted for the FKE approach, the predicted result for the UTD-PO approach indicates a significant improvement of 1.4873 dB. Also, data analysis for the two knife edge obstacles shows that UTD-PO approach gives a better result than the FKE approach.

Figure 6.12 shows a prediction of path loss over the multiple knife-edge obstacles where transmitter T_x of height h_{tx} of 46.42 λ is above the first obstacle height h_{obt1} of 42.41 λ and it is placed 86.06 λ away from the first obstacle. The second obstacle is of height h_{obt2} of 17.0 λ placed 17.08 λ away from the first obstacle. The third obstacle of height h_{obt3} of 46.50 λ is placed 12.91 λ away from the second obstacle. The receiver R_x has been placed 76.08 λ away from the third obstacle in the shadowed region. Propagation path loss is predicted when the receiver moves from *NLOS* to *LOS* vertically. The path loss results obtained for the UTD-PO and the FKE approaches show the same results when compared with the measurement data available for multiple knife-edge obstacles. Table 6.1 shows that the estimated path loss results obtained for the UTD-PO and the FKE approaches had mean errors of 1.3379 dB and 3.596 dB, respectively. When compared to the mean error result predicted for the FKE approach, the predicted result for the UTD-PO approach indicates a significant improvement of 2.2581 dB. Also, data analysis for multiple knife-edge obstacles shows that the UTD-PO approach gives a better result than the FKE approach. The above results also show

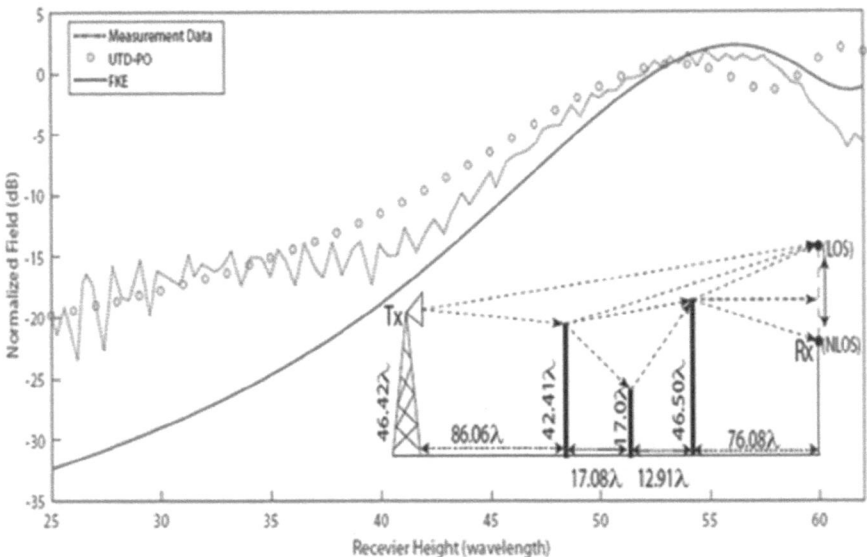

FIGURE 6.12　A comparison of the path loss obtained for multiple knife edge obstacles using the UTD-PO and the FKE approaches with the available measurement data.

TABLE 6.1
Mean Error (in dB)

Mean Error (in dB)	UTD-PO Approach	FKE Approach	UTD-PO show improvement over FKE
Figure 6.9	0.6443	0.6445	0.0002
Figure 6.10	0.2647	0.2648	0.0001
Figure 6.11	1.2192	2.7065	1.4873
Figure 6.12	1.3379	3.596	2.2581

that when the number of obstacles between transmitting and receiving points is one the UTD-PO and the FKE approaches give the same result. But when the number obstacles are increased, the path loss result for the FKE approach gives an inferior result than the path loss result obtained from the UTD-PO approach. This shows that the UTD-PO method is more accurate for predicting path loss over multiple obstacles, namely, the irregular terrain scenario.

6.4　CONCLUSION

In this work, the UTD-PO and the FKE approaches are studied to predict the path loss over an irregular terrain scenario. This scenario is a series of obstacles or hills of uneven height and spacing which is approximated as knife edge obstacles to predict path loss between transmitting and receiving points. The results of these scenarios show that when the path loss is predicted for one obstacle between the transmitting and the receiving point, both the approaches give exactly same results. But when the number of obstacles is increased to more than one, path loss for the FKE approach gives inferior results when compared with the path loss of measurement data and the path loss of the UTD-PO approach. Also, data analysis shows that the mean error for both the approaches in the case of one obstacle is same, but when the number of obstacles is more than one, the mean error of the UTD-PO approach is smaller than the mean error of the FKE approach. These results show that the predictions of path loss through the UTD-PO approach over a multiple obstacle scenario gives more accurate results than the FKE approach.

REFERENCES

1. Rodríguez, J. V. *et al.* A new solution for the analysis of multiple-building diffraction in urban areas with shadowing caused by a cylindrical hill. *IEEE Transactionon Antennas and Propagation* 55(9): 2632–2636, 2007.

2. Durkins Computer Prediction of Service Areas for VHF and UHF Land Mobile Radio Service. *IEEE Trans. Veh. Technol.* 26(4): 323–327, 1997.

3. Leubbers, R. J. Finite Conductivity uniform GTD versus Knife Edge Diffraction Prediction of Propagation Path Loss. *IEEE Trans. Antennas Propagat.* A32: 70–76, 1984.

4. Eliades, D. E. Terrain Simulation for the Cascadeed Cylinder Diffraction Model. *IEE Proceeding-H* 140(4): 285–291, 1993.

5. Luebbers, R. J. Propagation Prediction for Hilly Terrain Using GTD Wedge Diffraction. *IEEE Trans. Antennas Propagat.* AP- 32(9): 951–955, 1984.

6. Parson, J. D. *The Mobile Radio Propagation Channel.* edition 2nd. John Willey & Sons Ltd, 2000.

7. Kasampalis, S., and Lazaridis, P. *et al.* Longley-Rice Model Prediction Inaccuracies in the UHF and VHF TV bands in mountainous terrain. *IEEE BMSB ,* 2015.

8. Haung, K., and Qin, W. Improving the Computional Accuracy of RADAR Propagation Prediction Algorithm based on Digitized Terrain Elevation Data. *iWEM 201,* 1–3, 2016.

9. Topcu, S., and Goktas, P., *et al.* A New Approach to Diffraction Modelling for Line-of-Sight (LOS) Paths. *IEEE-APS Topical Conf. on APWC,* 696–699, 2015.

10. Lee, W. C. Y. *Mobile Communication Engineering.* edition 2nd. McGraw-Hill Educations, 2008.

11. Tzaras, C., and Saunders, S. R. Comparison of Multiple-Diffraction Models for Digital Broadcasting Coverage Prediction. *IEEE Trans. on Broadcasting* 46(3): 221–226, 2000.

12. Bertoni, H. L. *Radio Propagation for Modern Wireless Systems.* edition 2nd. Pearson Education Ltd, 2000.

13. Rappaprt,T. S. *Wireless Communication: Principles and Practice.* edition 2nd. PHI Pvt. Ltd, 2002.

14. Bertoni, H. L. *et al.* A theoretical model of UHF propagation in urban environments. *IEEE Transaction on Antennas and Propagation* 36(12): 1788–1796, 1988.

15. Saunders, S. R., and Bonar, F. R. Explicit multiple-building diffraction attenuation function for mobile radio wave propagation. *Electronic Letter* 27(14): 1276–1277, 1991.

16. Saunders, S. R., and Bonar, F. R. Prediction of mobile radio wave propagation over buildings of irregular heights and spacings. *IEEE Transaction on Antennas and Propagation* 42(2): 137–144, 1994.

17. Crosby, D. *et al.* The effect of building height variation on the multiplediffraction loss component of the Walfisch-Bertoni model. *In 14th IEEE 2003 international symposium on personal, indoor and mobile radio communication proceedings* 2: 1805–1809, 2003.

18. Tzaras, C., and Saunders, S. R. An improved heuristic UTD solution for multiple-edge transitionzone diffraction. *IEEE Transaction on Antennas and Propagation* 49(12): 1678–1682, 2001.

19. Koutitas, G., and Tzaras, C. A slope UTD solution for a cascade of multishaped canonical objects. *IEEE Transaction on Antennas and Propagation.* 54(10): 2969–2976, 2006.

20. Rodríguez, J. V. *et al.* A hybrid UTD-PO solution for multiple-cylinder diffraction analysis assuming spherical-wave incidence. *IEEE Transaction on Antennas and Propagation* 56(9): 3078–3081, 2008.

21. Rodríguez, J. V. *et al.* UTD-PO formulation for the multiple-diffraction of spherical waves by an array of multimodeled obstacles. *IEEE Antennas and Wireless Propagation Letters* 8: 379–382, 2009.

22. Erricolo, D., and D'Elia, G. Measurements on scaled models of urban environments and comparisons with ray-tracing propagation simulation. *IEEE Transaction on Antennas and Propagation* 50(5): 727–735, 2002.

23. Kumar, A., Albreem, M. A., Gupta, M. et. al. "Future 5G network based smart hospitals: Hybrid detection technique for latency improvement", IEEE Access, Vol 8, pp 153240–153249, 2020.

24. Kumar, A., Gupta, M., Le, D-N., Aly, A. A. "PTS-PAPR reduction technique for 5G advanced waveforms using BFO algorithm", Intelligent Automation and Soft Computing, Vol 27, No.3, pp 713–722, 2021.

25. Meena, K., Gupta, M., Kumar, A. "Analysis of UWB indoor and outdoor channel propagation", 2020 IEEE International Women in Engineering (WIE) Conference on Electrical and Computer Engineering (WIECON-ECE), pp 352–355, 2020.

26. Gupta, M., Chand, L. Pareek, M. "Power preservation in OFDM using selected mapping (SLM)", Journal of Statistics and Management Systems, Vol 22, No.4, pp 763–771, 2019.

27. Saeed, M., Hasan, M. K., Hassan, R. et. al. "Preserving privacy of user identity based on pseudonym variable in 5G" Computers, Materials & Continua, Vol.70, No.3, pp5551–5568, 2022.

29. Adarsh, A., Kumar, B., Gupta, M., Kumar, A. et. al. "Design of an Efficient Cooperative Spectrum for Intra-Hospital Cognitive Radio Network" Computers, Materials & Continua, Vol.69, No.1, pp 35–49, 2021.

29. Kumar, A., Gupta, M., Sharma, M. K. et. al. "Role of Detection Techniques in Mobile Communication for Enhancing the Performance of Remote Health Monitoring" Cyber-Physical Systems and Industry 4.0, Apple Cacdemic Press, pp 199–224, 2022.

30. Ranjan, P., Jhariya, D. K., Gupta, M. et.al. "Next-Generation Antennas:Advances and Challenges" Wiley Scrivener Publisher, pp 1–298, 2021.

7 Integrated Blockchain and MEC Systems Empower Healthcare Services

Amira A. Amer and Tawfik Ismail

CONTENTS

7.1 INTRODUCTION

Current healthcare application trends focus on providing quality healthcare services remotely through the medical Internet of Things (IoT) devices. The recent

COVID-19 crisis emphasized the importance of such telemedicine solutions. Recent reports estimate that the number of connected medical monitoring devices will increase to 83.4 million in 2023 and expects the global market size of the Internet of Things (IoT) in healthcare to rise to 188.2 billion USD by 2025 [1, 2]. Supporting several such devices can be achieved by integrating IoT devices with the emerging 5G networks.

Remote surgery and supplying remote assistance to paramedics in ambulances are examples of remote healthcare applications that require low latency response due to their criticality. For example, delay is a major performance measure for remote surgery since a delay of a mere second may case a patient's death. Aiding visuals and haptic feedback (for example, controlling a robotic arm and receiving feedback from sensors attached to the arm) expect an end-to-end delay of 10 ms and 1 ms respectively [3]. Deviating from the expected delay may cause cyber-sickness to surgeons and increase the surgery error rate [4]. 5G integrated with cloud computing alone cannot meet the latency requirements because the cloud infrastructure is located away from the end-users. Mobile edge computing (MEC) is a network architecture that provides computing and storage at the edge of the network so that computations are physically closer to the users. Adopting MEC architecture in 5G networks will enable 5G to support services with strict latency requirements.

A Stanford medical white paper estimated that 2,314 exabytes of healthcare data would be produced in 2020 and predicted that the annual increase in healthcare data would be at least 48% [5]. Such large amounts of data can also raise many privacy issues, making data security a primary concern for any organization. Healthcare IoT security issues have been growing in recent years as it is becoming clear that IoT devices are unsafe. This is primarily because most IoT devices and applications are not designed to handle security and privacy attacks. The blockchain is a promising cryptographic technology that could protect against data tampering. It could be able to address some of the challenges presented by healthcare IoT security. Moreover, the integration between AI and the blockchain will be more effective than those offered if only the blockchain is used.

7.1.1 MOTIVATION AND CONTRIBUTION

The increase of the aging population has pushed the need for Healthcare 4.0 systems that add automation to healthcare and allow doctors to perform their work remotely. To realize Healthcare 4.0, the needs of the new applications should be matched with capabilities of emerging telecommunication technologies and new computing paradigms. This chapter aims to explore the possible uses of different technologies for healthcare applications. Our contributions are as follows:

1. We introduce 5G enabling technologies and blockchain technology to readers and explore how each technology can support healthcare applications. Furthermore, we explore the challenges facing these technologies and give a brief survey on the attempt at solving these problems in literature.

2. We discuss the potential of integrating edge computing and blockchain and how this integration can shape healthcare applications. We also discuss the current state, results, and challenges of this integration.
3. We identify some future research opportunities that could enhance the performance of a healthcare system and add more automation to the system.
4. We present a case study to illustrate how new technologies could support healthcare applications.

These points are not all covered in previous works. In [6], Healthcare 4.0 applications and enabling devices are explored and the role of edge computing in decreasing computation latency is discussed, but no other technologies are mentioned. Qadri et al. [7] introduced edge computing, blockchains, machine learning and big data for healthcare. They discussed the current state and challenges of each technology, however a scenario where all technologies work together is not given. Moreover, the current state of the integration between these technologies is not explored.

7.2   ENABLING TECHNOLOGIES FOR HEALTHCARE IN 5G

The uses of 5G are classified by most of the requirements into three categories: enhanced mobile broadband (eMBB), massive machine-type communications (mMTC), and ultra-reliable low latency communications (URLLC). EMBB is designed to serve traffic with exceptionally high data rates (up to 10 Gbps) and large payloads of remote treatment using 3D videos. URLLC supports mission-critical applications with low latency requirements (about 1–10 ms) and requires reliable transmissions, such as remote surgery. MMTC is used for high-density connections (about 1 000 000 devices per square kilometer) from low-transmission devices, such as health monitoring devices. As mentioned above, MEC is a key technology to meet the latency requirements of URLLC services. 5G can also accommodate a range of services from different sectors that could be offered by network slicing.

7.2.1   NETWORK SLICING

The concept of network slicing has been introduced in 5G networks to support the different quality of service (QoS) requirements for each service type. Network slicing creates several logical networks, each designed to meet a specific requirement. Each slice of the network consists of virtual network functions and resources over the existing telecommunications infrastructure. Figure 7.1 demonstrates the concept of 5G network slicing.

The main issue with slicing is what should define a group of services to be in one slice. One approach is to have three slices that correspond to the service categories in 5G, an eMBB slice, an mMTC slice, and a URLLC slice. The problem with this technique is that some applications have specifications that cannot be fulfilled by one of the three slices alone. For example, remote surgery needs a highly reliable and low latency connection to reflect the controls done by the surgeon on the robotic arms. Simultaneously, the surgeon needs a high-quality 3D view of what happens at the

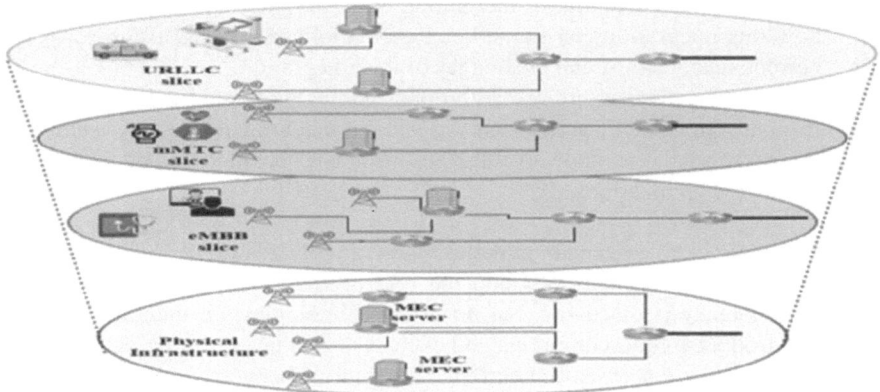

FIGURE 7.1 Network slicing in 5G.

remote site, which requires high data rates. One solution to this problem is expanding the slices to include a slice specifically for remote surgery. This approach of horizontally expanding slices according to need of the cases is not efficient. The maximum number of slices possible is 256, which could not fit all special use cases from all industries. A better approach is to slice according to latency, reliability, connection density, mobility, and security requirements. In this case, all applications requiring low latency, high reliability, low mobility, high security, and a low connection density demand will use the same slice. In case healthcare applications require any extra processing, the slice differentiator (SD) field specified in the 3GPP Release 15 specification [8] could be used. The SD is used to differentiate between tenants with the same slice number to provide each tenant with customized processing if needed.

7.2.2   MOBILE EDGE COMPUTING

Mobile edge computing is an architecture that provides computing capabilities within the network of radio accesses, as shown in Figure 7.2. Pushing cloud services to MEC servers near the access network decreases response latency and improves user experience. In order to satisfy the strict QoS criteria for some services, 5G networks will benefit from MEC technology.

Healthcare IoT devices have limited computing capabilities and cannot run demanding algorithms such as seizure detection algorithms. In MEC architecture, healthcare devices can offload the task of seizure detection to a MEC server. Offloading a task to the MEC server rather than the cloud has the advantage of sending an alert faster to the nearest hospital in case a seizure is detected. Offloading can also be used even if the healthcare device has enough computational power to save the devices' energy and reduce task latency. Power saving is significant for healthcare IoT devices that must have a long lifetime. This meets the goals of 5G networks in providing a better user experience and decreasing the energy consumption of services. MEC servers can also be used for aggregating and preprocessing data coming from

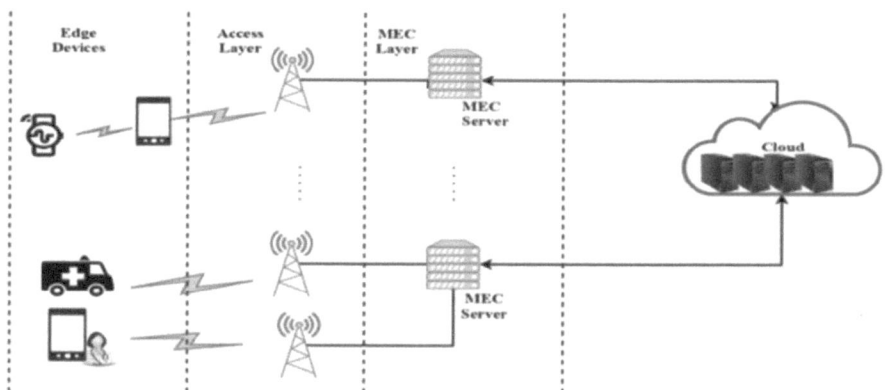

FIGURE 7.2   MEC architecture.

several healthcare sensors. Aggregation of sensor data can provide more insightful analytics about each patient. Furthermore, aggregation and preprocessing of data at MEC servers reduces the size of data added to the patient record on the cloud, which reduces the traffic on the telemedicine network. The storage on MEC servers can be used to cache records of patients who have appointments to be retrieved faster by the doctors.

7.3   THE BLOCKCHAIN IN HEALTHCARE

The blockchain is a distributed ledger technology that could provide a simple infrastructure for multiple devices to transfer data directly between them using a secure and reliable mechanism. Healthcare IoT applications require high protection to protect the privacy of each patient and prevent tampering with the data collected. The ability to provide a safe exchange of data in a public setting makes the blockchain a perfect candidate for IoT healthcare applications.

7.3.1   BLOCKCHAIN OVERVIEW

The blockchain is a sequence of connected blocks where each block records many transactions. Each block has a hash pointing to the previous block forming a blockchain, as shown in Figure 7.3. A block also has a timestamp and a Merkle tree root, a tree hash containing all transactions [9]. All the nodes on the network carry a replica of the whole blockchain. The blockchain structure renders it resistant to tampering. Any modifications to the existing block must change the hash of the block, causing the chain to be invalid. Also, any modifications to a current or new block will cause the root of the Merkle tree to be invalid. Even if the whole chain on one node is tampered with, this would be easily detected since the new chain does not match the replicas found on the other nodes. In this way, medical information can be exchanged among medical facilities without the possibility of being tampered with.

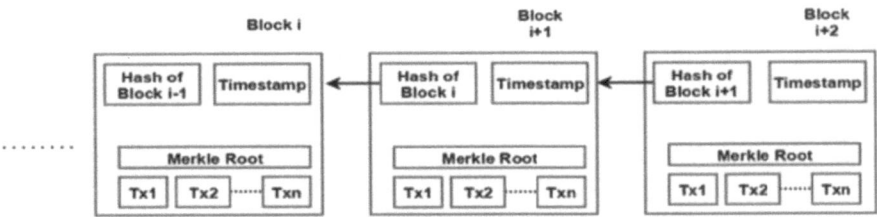

FIGURE 7.3   Blockchain architecture.

Another feature of blockchain technology is the validation of the transaction source. All transactions have a digital signature created using the author's private key. Other users can verify that the author of the transaction uses the author's public key. This function is essential if we want to verify that a surgeon rather than an impostor gives the operating robot commands. In order to compensate for the lack of a centralized transaction verification mechanism, blockchain uses a consensus algorithm to verify blocks in a decentralized fashion. The main challenge in developing consensus algorithms is how to make the algorithm immune to the existence of malicious nodes in the network. The most used consensus algorithms are job proof (PoW), stake proof (PoS), and practical byzantine fault tolerance (PBFT) [9].

7.3.2   SMART CONTRACTS AND AI

Smart contracts are scripts stored in the blockchain and have a unique address. The script is executed when a transaction addresses the smart contract [10]. Smart contracts resemble legal contracts where a transaction is not completed until all parties meet the conditions set in the contract. Smart contracts could be used to check that the medical personnel are authorized to edit a patient's record before appending new data to the record.

Artificial intelligence (AI) can expand the functionalities of blockchain and increase the security of blockchains. AI could detect anomalous readings from healthcare IoT sensors and discard them, which reduces the load on the blockchain network and makes the data used cleaner. AI can also be used to improve the efficiency of consensus algorithms by detecting malicious nodes. Moreover, integrating smart contracts with AI can expand the capabilities of smart contracts beyond if-else conditions. Smart contracts backed with AI can fulfill the automation expected from healthcare IoT applications. For example, AI-powered smart contracts can automatically notify a doctor if his patient is having a seizure and automatically records the event in the patient's record.

7.4   INTEGRATED BLOCKCHAIN AND MEC

Privacy and security of data is an essential requirement for all healthcare applications. Integrating blockchain and healthcare IoT networks makes the data more secure since it is stored in an encrypted block. Encrypting blocks and storing the blockchain requires computation capabilities not found in most healthcare IoT devices. Therefore, the data does not get encrypted until it reaches the cloud. Edge computing provides an early station where data could get encrypted. On the other hand, MEC lacks a secure mechanism to share sensitive data such as patient records among MEC nodes. Integrating blockchain and MEC with healthcare applications can increase the security level to the level required by healthcare applications. Blockchain can provide MEC with a secure method to share user requests and patient records among MEC nodes. MEC servers will provide an early point where healthcare sensor data and analytics can be encrypted.

Since a limited number of operators own the MEC nodes within one country, the blockchain network between MEC servers does not need to be public. A consortium blockchain could instead be used for the MEC network. Consortium blockchains are semi-private blockchains where a group of known entities has access to the network. The advantage of consortium blockchains is a less complicated consensus algorithm because the limited access on the blockchain means fewer chances of malicious nodes. The simplicity of consensus and the low latency provided by the MEC network can make the blockchain more scalable. This means that the blockchain can handle more transactions per unit time to cope with traffic generated by healthcare IoT devices.

Integration with blockchains can be used beyond security enhancement. AI-powered smart contracts can be used on edge to provide low latency process automation for emergency applications in healthcare IoT networks. For example, suppose a disaster is detected by analyzing data from various sensors. In that case, a notification can be sent automatically to all hospitals in the area to send aid and prepare for receiving emergency cases.

7.4.1 EXISTING WORK ON INTEGRATING BLOCKCHAIN AND MEC

Due to the complexity of implementing an integrated MEC and blockchain systems, most work is theoretical. Few projects have built a prototype for the system or part of the system to test their architecture and algorithms. Previous projects had different architectures for where the blockchain can be used. A blockchain can be placed on the cloud, the edge, or between devices in an IoT network or a combination of all of these. Guo et al. [11] suggested using blockchain on edge for authentication while the transaction recording is done on a blockchain on the cloud. Permission management can be placed instead in the cloud, as the case with MedRec [12]. Seng et al. [13] suggested a blockchain that connects end devices and MEC servers altogether.

The blockchain was used for sharing offloading tasks to other devices and the MEC server to decide where best to place the task in a decentralized manner. Results showed that their solution reached a better offloading success rate and less energy consumption compared to centralized offloading techniques. However, there is no analysis for the latency of their framework compared to the centralized approach. EdgeBot [14] uses a 4-layer architecture, namely, the sensor, edge, fog, and cloud layers. The blockchain and smart contracts are hosted at the fog layer, which manages several edge gateways. Edge gateways collect and analyze data and send it to the fog layer. The fog layer acts as a data gatekeeper between data from sensors and the cloud applications requesting the data. This way, only authorized entities can send or receive data. EdgeMediChain [15] breaks down the blockchain into two parts for more efficiency. The first part is the local edge-mining layer which manages the authentication of IoT devices within their geolocation without downloading information about users outside their range. Local edge-mining layers reach consensus about their state through proof-of-authority (PoA), which does not require computationally intensive work. The second part is the global blockchain, based on Ethereum, which contains hashes of transactions done on the EMR of all patients. The EMR itself is stored on InterPlanetary File System (IPFS). To decrease the global blockchain burden, the local edge sends data to the global blockchain only when an event occurs.

7.4.2 BLOCKCHAIN AND MEC INTEGRATION RESULTS

To assess the solutions proposed, we compare the result from two different works based on execution time and scalability. One work is Hyperledger Fabric based [14], and the other is Ethereum based [15]. Figure 7.4 shows the execution time taken for a task in each framework in milliseconds, and Figure 7.5 shows the number of transactions per second supported by each system. Both results are obtained for a setting with 400 clients.

The results show that EdgeBot is faster compared to EdgeMediChain, which can be because Hyperledger Fabric and Ethereum have different latencies. Since Hyperledger Fabric is a permissioned blockchain, less complicated algorithms could authorize transactions than a permissionless blockchain such as Ethereum. On the other side, EdgeMediChain can support many more transactions per second due to having a local edge-mining layer that filters out data that will not create a useful transaction and makes the authorization of devices easier. Given the permissioned nature of Hyperledger Fabric, it would be challenging to have such a system to authorize an ever-increasing number of devices and users. However, it could still be used to connect edge nodes or cloud servers as they are less likely to change. As shown by the results of EdgeMediChain, more thought should be given to the system architecture and how to take advantage of different technologies, making the system faster and more scalable.

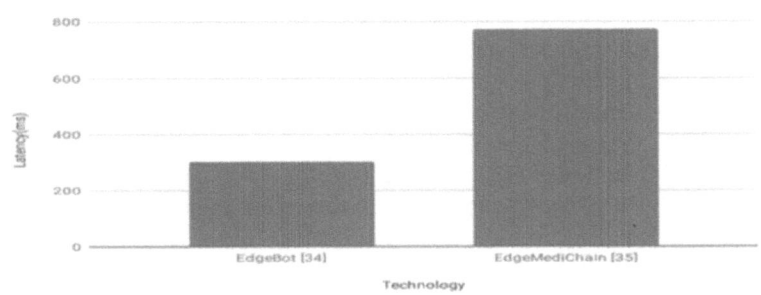

FIGURE 7.4   Execution time in EdgeBot vs EdgeMediChain.

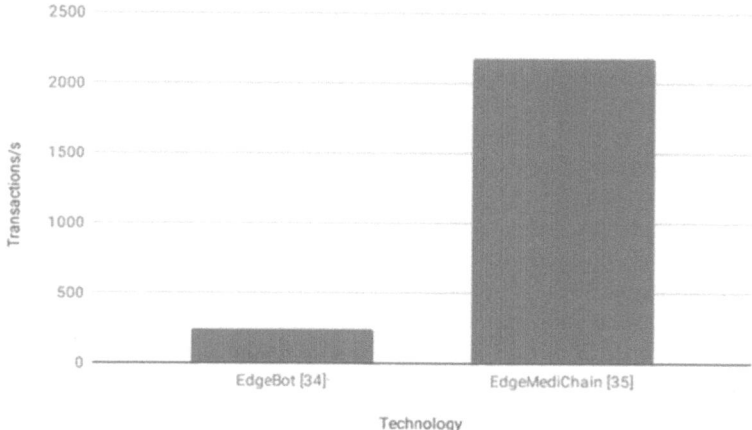

FIGURE 7.5   Scalability of EdgeBot vs EdgeMediChain.

7.5   RESEARCH OPPORTUNITIES AND THE CHALLENGES OF HEALTHCARE

Although 5G and blockchain show a great promise in supporting healthcare applications, we must address open issues in each to reach the full potential of these technologies. This section highlights the main issues and discusses possible solutions for 5G and blockchain in healthcare applications.

7.5.1   RESOURCE ALLOCATION CHALLENGE

Computational and QoS requirements for each request need to be allocated physical resources that fulfill both requirements. The decision on where to place the task is the responsibility of the network orchestrator. The orchestrator may allocate computational resources on MEC servers or the cloud according to the availability of resources on MEC servers and on QoS requirements. Furthermore, other factors, such as task priority and energy consumption, can affect the allocation. Task priority implies how critical the task is, and therefore blocking high-priority tasks should be minimized. Minimizing energy consumption is an important factor to consider, especially since the power capabilities of healthcare IoT devices are limited.

Orchestrator architectures can be classified as centralized, such as in [16–18], or decentralized, such as in [19, 20]. Centralized orchestrators are typically placed as cluster heads for a group of base stations or at the core network. In this architecture, the orchestrator receives requests from several base stations and decides which MEC server they should be allocated to or whether the cloud best serves their requests. In the case of a decentralized orchestrator, the allocation decision is taken collaboratively by MEC servers. Each server broadcasts its status to the other servers in the network so that no server is overloaded, and the total number of requests satisfied is maximized. The advantage of using centralized orchestration is that it manages requests and balances network loads easily, transfers less data over the network, and can be implemented over the current infrastructure with simple modifications. The problem with centralized orchestrators is a single point of failure. The decentralized architecture eliminates the single point of failure but overloads the network with a broadcasting status message from one node to its neighbors.

Both centralized and decentralized orchestrators use a decision-making approach to reach the best solution to the multi-objective resource allocation problem. Optimization techniques use algorithms that minimize a mathematical function that represents the given problem. Optimization techniques used for resource allocation include genetic algorithms [19–21], greedy algorithms [18], and the iterative search algorithm [22]. In game-theoretic methods, the problem is modeled as a game where each user device or MEC server is a player, and the goal is to reach a Nash equilibrium state. Nash equilibrium is a state where each player cannot decrease their overhead by changing their chosen strategy. To reach the Nash equilibrium, each player considers the equilibrium offloading strategy of other players and tries to choose an offloading strategy that decreases the computation and delay overhead. The conflict graphs used in [21] is an example of using graph theory in resource allocation. In this approach, nodes represent possible assignments for each task, and edges represent conflicts between assignments. Each node holds the cost of the assignment, and a minimum weighted vertex search algorithm is used to find the best assignment that has no conflicts. Deep reinforcement learning (DRL) was proposed as a resource allocation technique by Luong et al. [23] because it can provide autonomous decision-making and considers long-term reward. Most DRL techniques use deep Q networks [24, 25] or their variant, the double-Q [26].

All methods consider one or more of the following factors to decide the best assignment:

1. Task delay on MEC versus cloud (includes the processing delay plus the propagation delay)
2. Energy consumed by assigning task on MEC versus cloud (includes the processing energy consumption+ transmission energy consumption)
3. Monetary cost of assigning task on MEC versus cloud.

Minimizing these factors is constrained by the maximum delay allowed for each task and the resources available on MEC servers. Task priority can be considered by adding a violation penalty that corresponds to the priority of the task. Therefore, assignments that cause high priority violations will have a higher cost and will be eliminated.

7.5.2 Mobility Challenge

Indoor health monitoring sensors are one example of low mobility healthcare applications. A 5G connected ambulance is an example of high mobility healthcare applications. Like older mobile network generations, 5G should effectively associate an end-user with the most appropriate access point and handle handovers. An extra parameter to consider in MEC is how will resource allocation algorithms handle handovers. The higher the mobility, the more challenging it is to allocate resources that fulfill the QoS requirements of each request.

To solve the network association problem, Zhu et al. [27] propose a network selection scheme using decision theory and fuzzy logic theory. They base their decision on the QoS required by the user, the cost of associating with the network, and the network load. For mobility aware resource allocation, two methods were mentioned in [28]. One method is to provide the orchestrator with real-time user information to predict the user location and consider it to decide the allocation. The other method is to reserve resources on each server to improve the scheduling of tasks that migrate from one edge node to another. The main concern with the task migration method is that it induces unnecessary communication overhead in a false handover alarm. The interesting idea is to build two different protocols for dealing with network association and resource allocation. Low mobility applications will follow one protocol, whereas the other protocol focuses on solving serious mobility application problems. Network slicing can be used to categorize the request and determine the protocol that should be used.

7.5.3 PROBLEMS AND CHALLENGES IN INTEGRATION

7.5.3.1 Scalability

In blockchain systems, scalability is defined by the number of transactions per second. Scalability is governed by the speed of consensus and the block size. Currently used consensus mechanisms require verification from more than one node. A limit is placed on the block size to speed up the exchange of transactions for verification. Even with a limit placed on the transaction, a consensus is considered slow compared to speeds required in Healthcare 4.0 applications. Waiting for consensus before propagating alerts and timely information destroys this information's purpose and may lead to failing in the QoS of the required task. Methods to increase transaction speed should be explored to benefit from the integration between blockchain and edge fully.

Due to the limited transaction size, storing large files, such as electronic health records (EHR), is challenging on a blockchain. To secure these files off the blockchain, MedRec [12] uses a blockchain for permission management of the patient's medical history. A smart contract for each authorized person is present to record data entered by this person in the EHR database. A hash of the data is saved in the blockchain to allow database auditing. The problem with the MedRec approach is that the data is stored in a centralized location which puts the cloud in control of the data rather than the patient. To overcome centralization, authors in [29] used IPFS for storage while keeping the blockchain as a source for permission management.

7.5.3.2 Identity Management in a Mobile Scenario

In remote control and autonomous applications, such as remote surgery and self-driving ambulances, verifying the source of control is important. A local blockchain connecting the access point and end devices can enhance the data source authentication [30]. Local blockchains might be a good solution for static or low mobility devices, as surgery robots, that don't change their access points often. Mobile devices, such as ambulances, need to exchange keys with every access point as they hand over which could be an overhead on both the network and the device.

7.5.3.3 Security Challenge

Although blockchain boosts the security of MEC networks, they are not immune to attacks by quantum computers. Current cryptography methods used in blockchain are easily breakable by quantum computing. Quantum key distribution methods can be used to improve the resistance to quantum computing attacks.

As an open system, MEC is vulnerable to distributed denial-of-service (DDoS) attacks. Blockchain cannot provide immunity to such types of attack. DDoS attacks overload the MEC servers and decrease the probability of satisfying the QoS of customers. Orchestrators should be provided with AI algorithms to predict DDoS attacks and detect malicious users to deny their access to the resources.

7.6 RESEARCH OPPORTUNITIES: BLOCKCHAIN AND EDGE COMPUTING IN HEALTHCARE

7.6.1 ENSEMBLE LEARNING AND BLOCKCHAIN FOR DECISION-MAKING

Ensemble learning combines predictions from different machine learning to get more accurate results. Ensemble learning has proved to have a superior performance in various fields, including healthcare [31]. Edge could use predictions from end devices and sensor analytics in an ensemble model to send a more reliable diagnosis to the cloud and decrease the chances of sounding false alarms. A more interesting scenario is an emergency response in a smart city where the protocol followed is decided by information from hospitals, environment or factory sensors, wearables, and police. Each entity may send its data on a different MEC server, and data shared across these entities is restricted to protecting each entity's privacy. Decisions can be made by the MEC server using ensemble learning on predictions and information sent from each entity. Therefore, actions are taken autonomously without the need to share data across entities.

In their current form, blockchain can record transactions that all nodes can verify. This model is suitable for asset exchange but not for decision making, where each entity provides a different view on the same problem. Decision-making needs a way to share the decisions and information coming from different systems. Salman et al. [32] introduced a probabilistic blockchain model to support decision-making data, which can make secure emergency response systems realizable. Use cases for probabilistic blockchains still need to be explored and tested.

7.6.2 FEDERATED LEARNING

Machine learning models on MEC servers need to be continuously updated to cope with new data and become more personalized to the users it is serving. Traditionally, collected data is sent to the cloud to re-train the machine learning model and then update it on all MEC servers. This technique overloads the cloud and risks the security of data. Khan et al. [33] suggested using federated learning between edge nodes to overcome centralized model update downsides. In federated learning, only the updated weights are shared, preserving data privacy, and decreasing the amount of data that needs to be shared. Implementing and orchestrating federated learning across MEC servers needs to be further studied. Also, the benefits of large-scale federated learning between MEC servers from different neighborhoods have not been studied.

7.7 CASE STUDY: REAL-TIME PATIENT MONITORING

One aspect of Healthcare 4.0 is real-time monitoring, which aims to improve healthcare systems by providing real-time patient data and using AI for diagnosis, analytics, and decision-making [34]. Real-time monitoring includes raising alerts for any severe medical conditions, such as cardiac arrest. Raising early alerts can help patients get aid faster, increasing the survival chances of the patient. AI's diagnosis should also be added to the patient's electronic health records (EHR) automatically. Implementing a real-time monitoring system will increase the number of connected devices, increasing the traffic and the risk of patient data exposure. Furthermore, involved devices and users may use different technologies and may be supported by different operators. These challenges can only be satisfied through 5G networks that promise increased network capacity, interoperability, and security.

Edge computing could be used to do light analytics on data before sending the data for further processing and recording on the cloud. Early processing of data compresses the traffic going to the cloud, reducing congestion, and decreasing the cloud load. Furthermore, less patient data is transferred over the network, decreasing privacy leakage. AI detection models could also be deployed on edge to detect severe conditions within the edge layer. An alert can be issued to medical users in the neighborhood. Blockchain provides a secure channel to share data across different parties while disallowing unauthorized access and preserving patient privacy. Smart contracts could be used along with AI models to automatically record observations and diagnoses obtained from sensor data in the patient's EHR.

A full real-time emergency use case scenario is illustrated in Figure 7.6. Sensor data is sent to the nearest edge device. Data is passed to AI models on one of the MEC servers to be analyzed. Analyzed data is committed to the blockchain, which triggers a smart contract to add the patient record's new information. An alert is issued through a local blockchain that connects edge devices in the same neighborhood in case of an emergency. The alert is sent to the nearest emergency assistance system. As in [35], traffic systems are also given a notification to clear the way for an ambulance automatically. In this system, edge provides a low latency response to the emergency, and blockchain provides a channel to preserve the privacy of the patient's data and a secure method for MEC servers to share their knowledge and act.

7.8 CONCLUSION

Next-generation healthcare applications require networks to have higher security, lower latencies, and a method to deal with requests of different requirements. MEC and network slicing concepts allow 5G networks to support diverse and strict requirements

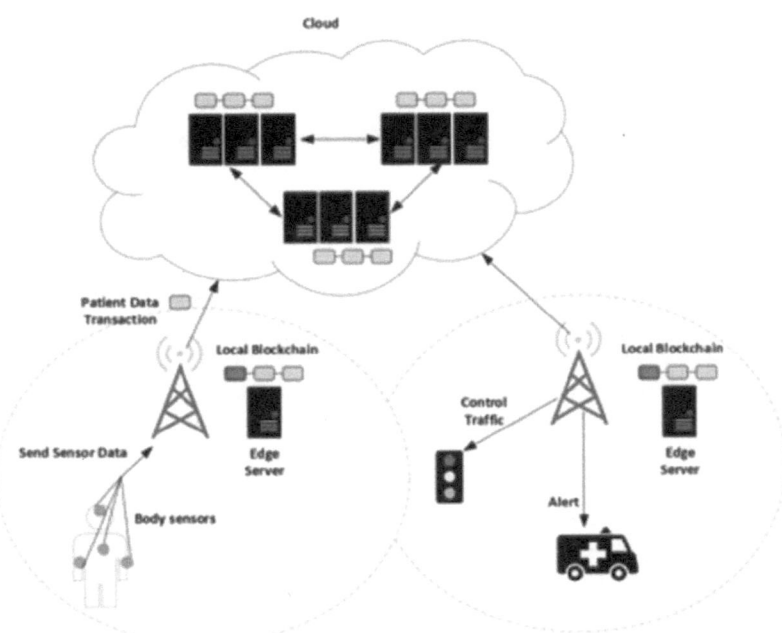

FIGURE 7.6   Blockchain and edge computing for remote patient monitoring.

in new healthcare technologies. MEC provides computation power at the network edge that decreases the latency of requests. However, MEC faces resource allocation and mobility issues that need solving to benefit from this technology. Some solutions found in the literature were discussed, but further study is still needed. Network slicing gives a solution to differentiate the requirements of the services to follow the best protocol for dealing with each request. Blockchain technology is key to supply both security and authentication required by healthcare applications.

Moreover, blockchain powered with AI smart contracts opens new opportunities in healthcare IoT applications. Integrating these technologies has a great potential for realizing Healthcare 4.0, as shown by the patient monitoring case study. Scalability and identity management issues of this integration should be solved to allow the realization of this system practically. Solving these issues will also allow further study of hosting federated learning and decision-making systems on edge securely.

REFERENCES

1. Rep. *MHealth and Home Monitoring – 9th Edition.* Berg Insight, December 2018.
2. Rep. IoT in Healthcare Market by Component (Medical Device, Systems and Software, Services, and Connectivity Technology), Application (Telemedicine, Connected Imaging, and Inpatient Monitoring), End User, and Region – Global Forecast to 2025. Markets and Markets, June 2020.

3. Gupta, R., Tanwar, S., Tyagi, S., and Kumar, N. "Tactile internet and its applications in 5G era: A comprehensive review." *International Journal of Communication Systems* 32, no. 14: e3981, 2019.

4. Wazid, M., Das, A. K., and Lee, J-H. "User authentication in a tactile internet based remote surgery environment: Security issues, challenges, and future research directions." *Pervasive and Mobile Computing* 54: 71–85, 2019.

5. Minor, Dean. Rep. Harnessing the Power of Data in Health. Stanford Medicine, 2017.

6. Singh, A. and Chatterjee, K. "Securing smart healthcare system with edge computing.", *Computers & Security* 108: 102353, September 2021.

7. Qadri, Y. A., Nauman, A., Zikria, Y. B., Vasilakos, A. V., and Kim, S. W. "The future of healthcare internet of things: A survey of emerging technologies." *IEEE Communications Surveys & Tutorials* 22, no. 2: 1121–1167, 2020.

8. 3GPP. Tech. System Architecture for the 5G System (3GPP TS 23.501 Version 15.3.0 Release 15), 2018.

9. Dai, H-N., Zheng, Z., and Zhang, Y. "Blockchain for Internet of Things: A survey." *IEEE Internet of Things Journal* 6, no. 5: 8076–8094, 2019.

10. Ali, M. S., Vecchio, M., Pincheira, M., Dolui, K., Antonelli, F., and Rehmani, M. H. "Applications of Blockchains in the Internet of Things: A Comprehensive Survey," *IEEE Communications Surveys & Tutorials*, vol. 21, no. 2: 1676–1717, Second Quarter 2019, doi: 10.1109/COMST.2018.2886932.

11. Guo, S., Hu, X., Guo, S., Qiu, X., and Qi, F. "Blockchain meets edge computing: A distributed and trusted authentication system." *IEEE Transactions on Industrial Informatics* 16, no. 3: 1972–1983, 2019.

12. Azaria, A., Ekblaw, A., Vieira, T., and Lippman, A. "Medrec: Using blockchain for medical data access and permission management." In 2016 2nd International Conference on Open and Big Data (OBD), pp. 25–30. IEEE, 2016.

13. Seng, S., Li, X, Luo, C., Ji, H., and Zhang, H. "A D2D-assisted MEC computation offloading in the blockchain-based framework for UDNs." In ICC 2019–2019 IEEE International Conference on Communications (ICC), pp. 1–6. IEEE, 2019.

14. Melo, W. S., Bessani, A., Neves, N., Santin, A. O., and Carmo, L. F. R. C. "Using blockchains to implement distributed measuring systems." *IEEE Transactions on Instrumentation and Measurement* 68, no. 5: 1503–1514, 2019.

15. Akkaoui, R., Hei, X., and Cheng, W. "EdgeMediChain: A hybrid edge blockchain-based framework for health data exchange." *IEEE Access* 8: 113467–113486, 2020.

16. Wang, J., Zhao, L., Liu, J., and Kato, N. "Smart resource allocation for mobile edge computing: A deep reinforcement learning approach." *IEEE Transactions on Emerging Topics in Computing*, vol. 9, no. 3: 1529–1541, 1 July–Sept. 2021, doi: 10.1109/ TETC.2019.2902661.

17. Skarlat, O., Nardelli, M., Schulte, S., Borkowski, M., and Leitner, P. "Optimized IoT service placement in the fog." *Service Oriented Computing and Applications* 11, no. 4: 427–443, 2017.

18. Yousefpour, A., Patil, A. Ishigaki, G., Kim, I., Wang, X., Cankaya, H. C., Zhang, Q., Xie, W., and Jue, J. P. "Fog Plan: a lightweight QoS-aware dynamic fog service provisioning framework." *IEEE Internet of Things Journal* 6, no. 3: 5080–5096, 2019.

19. Sahni, Y., Cao, J., Zhang, S., and Yang, L. "Edge mesh: A new paradigm to enable distributed intelligence in internet of things." *IEEE access* 5: 16441–16458, 2017.

20. Mahmud, R., Srirama, S. N., Ramamohanarao, K., and Buyya, R. "Quality of Experience (QoE)-aware placement of applications in Fog computing environments." *Journal of Parallel and Distributed Computing* 132: 190–203, 2019.

21. Al-Habob, A. A., Dobre, O. A., Armada, A. G., and Muhaidat, S. "Task scheduling for mobile edge computing using genetic algorithm and conflict graphs." *IEEE Transactions on Vehicular Technology*, vol. 69, no. 8: 8805–8819, Aug. 2020, doi: 10.1109/TVT.2020.2995146.

22. Zhang, J., Hu, X., Ning, Z., Ngai, E. C-H., Zhou, L, Wei, J., Cheng, J., and Hu, B. "Energy-latency tradeoff for energy-aware offloading in mobile edge computing networks." *IEEE Internet of Things Journal* 5, no. 4: 2633–2645, 2017.

23. Luong, N. C., Hoang, D. T., Gong, S. Niyato, D. Wang, P. Liang, Y.-C., and Kim, D. I. "Applications of deep reinforcement learning in communications and networking: A survey." *IEEE Communications Surveys & Tutorials* 21, no. 4: 3133–3174, 2019.

24. Wang, J., Zhao, L. Liu, J., and Kato, N. "Smart resource allocation for mobile edge computing: A deep reinforcement learning approach." *IEEE Transactions on Emerging Topics in Computing*, 2019.

25. Liu, Y., Yu, H., Xie, S., and Zhang, Y. "Deep reinforcement learning for offloading and resource allocation in vehicle edge computing and networks." *IEEE Transactions on Vehicular Technology* 68, no. 11: 11158–11168, 2019.

26. Zhao, N., Liang, Y-C. Niyato, D. Pei, Y., Wu, M., and Jiang, Y. "Deep reinforcement learning for user association and resource allocation in heterogeneous cellular networks." *IEEE Transactions on Wireless Communications* 18, no. 11: 5141–5152, 2019.

27. Zhu, A., Guo, S., Liu, B., Ma, M., Yao, J., and Su, X. "Adaptive multiservice heterogeneous network selection scheme in mobile edge computing." *IEEE Internet of Things Journal* 6, no. 4: 6862–6875, 2019.

28. Waqas, M., Niu, Y., Ahmed, M., Li, Y., Jin, D., and Han, Z. "Mobility-aware fog computing in dynamic environments: Understandings and implementation." *IEEE Access* 7: 38867–38879, 2018.

29. Sun, J., Yao, X., Wang, S., and Wu, Y. "Blockchain-based secure storage and access scheme for electronic medical records in IPFS." *IEEE Access* 8: 59389–59401, 2020.

30. Yang, R., Richard Yu, F., Si, P., Yang, Z., and Zhang, Y. "Integrated blockchain and edge computing systems: A survey, some research issues and challenges." *IEEE Communications Surveys & Tutorials* 21, no. 2: 1508–1532, 2019.

31. Pintelas, P., and Livieris, I. E. "Special issue on ensemble learning and applications": 140, 2020.

32. Salman, T., Jain, R., and Gupta, L. "Probabilistic blockchains: A blockchain paradigm for collaborative decision-making." In 2018 9th IEEE Annual Ubiquitous Computing, Electronics & Mobile Communication Conference (UEMCON), pp. 457–465. IEEE, 2018.

33. Khan, L. U., Yaqoob, I. Tran, N. H., Ahsan Kazmi, S.M., Dang, T. N., and Hong, C. S. "Edge-computing-enabled smart cities: A comprehensive survey." *IEEE Internet of Things Journal* 7, no. 10: 10200–10232, 2020.

34. Chanchaichujit, J., Tan, A., Meng, F., and Eaimkhong, S. "An introduction to healthcare 4.0." In *Healthcare 4.0*, pp. 1–15. Palgrave Pivot, Singapore, 2019.

35. Konstantinou, D., Rommel, S., Morales, A., Raddo, T. R., Johannsen, U., and Monroy, I. T. "An ehealth-care driven perspective on 5G networks and infrastructure." In *Interactive Mobile Communication, Technologies and Learning*, Michael E. Auer and Thrasyvoulos Tsiatsos (Eds.), pp. 1076–1088. Springer, Cham, 2019.

8 Optimized Cognitive Radio Networks for 5G Technology

Mohammed Ali Ahmed Alrefaei,
Ubaid M. Al-Saggaf, Muhammad Moinuddin,
and Asmaa U. Al-Saggaf

CONTENTS

8.1 INTRODUCTION

The rapid growth of wireless technologies with the limited frequency spectrum demands an intelligent utilization of electromagnetic spectrum resources [1].

The study in [2] shows that in the existing communication systems, only a small percentage of the spectrum is fully utilized. The rest of the spectrum is either mostly unutilized or underutilized as demonstrated in Figure 8.1.

More precisely, the fixed spectrum allocation policy is not capable of accommodating the unutilized portion of the spectrum, and this is the main reason behind the development of the CRN. The CRN enhances the efficient utilization of the spectrum allocated to any region by reusing the vacant frequency slots. This vacant frequency slot is termed "spectrum hole" as shown in Figure 8.2.

Spectrum hole is originally assigned to an absent licensed user, labeled the primary user (PU). The task of the CRN is to detect such spectrum holes and assign them to a non-licensed user in need, labeled the secondary user (SU). The SU can utilize

DOI: 10.1201/9781003368311-8

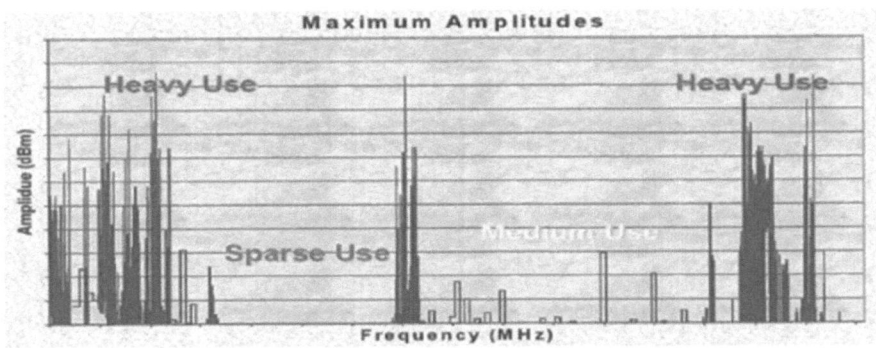

FIGURE 8.1   Power Spectrum of a typical communication system [2].

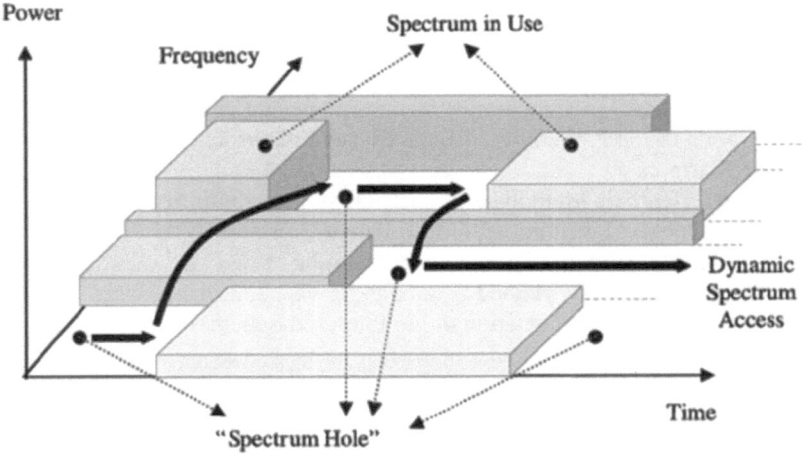

FIGURE 8.2   Illustration of Spectrum Holes [2].

that frequency band that otherwise PU keeps using its frequency. In summary, the CRN always gives priority to the PU over the SU, unless the spectrum is vacant [3].

There is a great interest in the development of an efficient spectrum-sensing method as it is the key process in any CRN. Various methods of spectrum sensing include energy-based detectors [4–9], which have low computational complexity and reasonably good performance. Thus, in this work, novel techniques for energy-detection (ED) based spectrum sensing methods are explored.

8.2   RELATED LITERATURE REVIEW

There is an amount of work in the literature, focusing on the spectrum sensing solutions for CRN. For instance, D. Cabric has developed spectrum sensing in a cross-layer design [10]. This work shows that among the three different detection methods proposed for spectrum sensing, the pilot detection method requires a minimum amount of sensing time at the expense of the perfect synchronization requirement. Moreover, it shows that the performance of the ED method is limited by the longest processing times the noise uncertainties. On the other hand, the ED methods are found to be better in a low signal-to-noise ratio (SNR) scenario [4–9].

The benefits of cooperation based spectrum sensing (CSS) in the CRN are illustrated in [11]. Specifically, it shows that cooperation within the same frequency band can reduce the detection time which in turn improves the overall processing time. Among the existing CSS schemes, the methods are broadly categorized into three fusion techniques: data-based fusion, hard decision-based fusion, and soft decision-based fusion [12]. In [13], it was shown that CSS parameters can be optimized by employing a likelihood ratio test (LRT).

In [14], different simpler CSS techniques are presented. Among these, the simplest method is the one that utilizes an OR operation [15]. Works in [16, 17] are based on the k-out-of-N fusion rule where the k value can be optimized.

In ED based SS under Rayleigh fading, various combining techniques are investigated which include equal gain combining, selection combining, and switch and stay combining [18].

For hard fusion in CSS, there are several methods such as AND [19], OR [19], M-out-of-N [20], and optimal linear combination [21]. In [22], the weights of linear cooperation are optimized to enhance the overall CSS performance.

In all the ED based SS techniques, the received signal energy is compared with a threshold value to decide the existence/absence of PU such that the probability of detection is maximized while the probability of a false alarm is maintained under some particular acceptable level. To do so, the precise choice of threshold value is also a challenge in the ED based SS methods [23]. For this purpose, there are various techniques to obtain a precise threshold value. One of the techniques is based on a constraint on the probability of a false alarm [23].

8.3   SYSTEM MODEL: NON-COOPERATIVE SPECTRUM SENSING IN THE CRN

Consider a non-cooperative spectrum sensing scenario where the local decision is made via processing of the PU signal by the energy detection method with respect to hypotheses H_o and H_1 as shown in Figure 8.3. It consists of a number of co-channels, C. Each SU is equipped with an $MX1$ antenna array.

Hypotheses H_0 shows the scenario where the ith node decides that the primary user is not available (absent) and is given by:

$$H_0 : x_{o,i}[t \mid H_o] = \sum_{c=1}^{c} \sqrt{E_{c,i}}\, h_{c,i}^{H} w x_{c,i}\left(t\right) + n_{o,i}\left(t\right) \tag{8.1}$$

Hypotheses H_1 shows the scenario when the ith node decides that the primary user is available (present) and is given by:

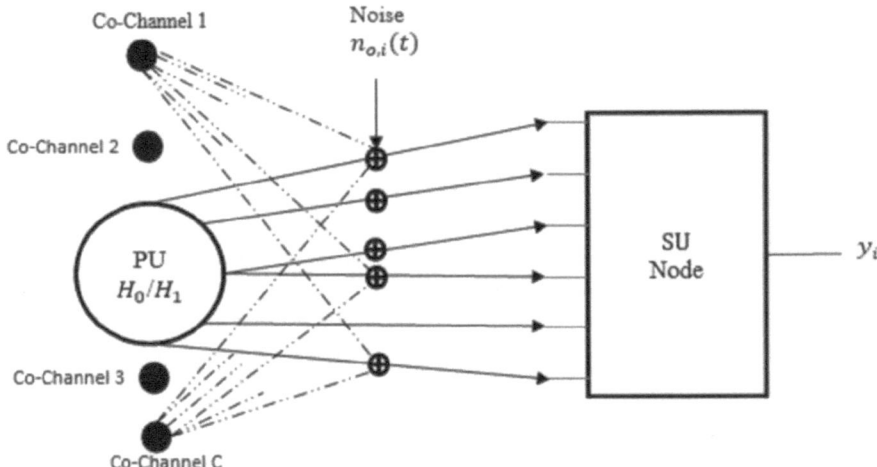

FIGURE 8.3 Architecture of the Beamforming-based Spectrum Sensing System Model.

$$H_1 : x_{o,i}[t \mid H_1] = \sqrt{E_o}\, h_{o,i}^H wx(t) + \sum_{c=1}^{c} \sqrt{E_{c,i}}\, h_{c,i}^H wx_{c,i}(t) + n_{o,i}(t) \qquad (8.2)$$

At each node, the received signal $x_{o,i}[t]$ is sampled with a rate of $f_s = 1/T_s$ Hz over a time duration of $\tau = NT_s$ s where T_s denotes the sampling period, and N denotes the number of samples that were utilized for the SS. The sampled version of the received signal is represented by $x_{o,i}[n]$ at discrete time n which can be expressed as:

$$x_{o,i}[n \mid H_o] = \sum_{c=1}^{c} \sqrt{E_{c,i}}\, h_{c,i}^H wx_{c,i}\left(nT_s\right) + n_{o,i}\left(nT_s\right)$$

$$x_{o,i}[n \mid H_1] = \sqrt{E_o}\, h_{o,i}^H wx\left(nT_s\right) + \sum_{c=1}^{c} \sqrt{E_{c,i}}\, h_{c,i}^H wx_{c,i}\left(nT_s\right) + n_{o,i}\left(nT_s\right)$$

In the above, the average transmitted symbol energy of the licensed user (PU) signal and the energy of the co-channel interferer (CCI) signal are denoted as (E_o/E_c) respectively. The square root of the symbol energy is multiplied with the Hermitian of the channel fading coefficient between a PU node and an SU node $h_{o,i}^H$. Also, the square root of the energy of the co-channel interferer is multiplied with the Hermitian of the channel fading coefficient between the ith CCI node and SU node $h_{c,i}^H$. $n_{o,i}(t)$ represents the sensing noise, assuming additive white Gaussian random variables with zero mean and variance σ_n^2 experiencing independently and identically distributed (i.i.d.) fading effects.

From the above two hypotheses, the distribution of the received signal at each antenna element is given below, where it is assumed to be an i.i.d. random process with complex normal distribution with zero mean and a correlation matrix defined below.

$$x_i \mid H_0 \sim \mathcal{CN}\left(0, R_{I+n}\right)$$

$$x_i \mid H_1 \sim \mathcal{CN}\left(0, R_{S+I+n}\right)$$

R_{I+n} is the correlation matrix of H_0 which represents the expectation of an interference term plus a sensing noise term.

$$R_{I+n} = E\left[(I+n)(I+n)^H\right] = R_{I+n} = E\left[II^*\right] + E\left[nn^*\right]$$

Because of the i.i.d. condition, we have $E\left[In^*\right] = E\left[nI^*\right] = 0$.
Using the trace properties, we can rewrite it as:

$$R_{I+n} = \sum_{c=1}^{c} E_c T_r E\left[h_c^H w w^H h_c\right] + \sigma_n^2$$

The expectation of a CCI channel vector multiplied by its Hermitian $E\left[h_c h_c^H\right]$ produces a correlation matrix of that channel vector (R_c).

$$R_{I+n} = \sum_{c=1}^{c} E_c T_r\left[R_c w w^H\right] + \sigma_n^2$$

Similarly, R_{S+I+n} is the correlation matrix of the received signal for H_1 which represents the expectation of a PU transmitted signal term plus an interference term plus a sensing noise term, multiplied by their conjugate transpose.
$R_{S+I+n} = R_S + R_{I+n}$, where the PU signal, interference, and noise are all independent.

$$R_{S+I+n} = E\left[SS^*\right] + E\left[II^*\right] + E\left[nn^*\right]$$

$$R_{S+I+n} = E_o E\left[\left(h_o^H w\right)\left(h_o^H w\right)^*\right] + R_{I+n}$$

Using trace properties, we can rewrite it as:

$$R_{S+I+n} = E_o T_r\left[h_o^H w w^H h_o\right] + \sigma_{H_0}^2$$

$$R_{S+I+n} = E_o T_r\left[R_o w w^H\right] + \sigma_{H_0}^2$$

The expectation of a PU channel multiplied by its Hermitian $E\left[h_o h_o^H\right]$ produces a correlation matrix of that channel (R_o). For the ED-based spectrum sensing in the CRN, the ith SU measures the average energy of the received signal as follows:

$$y_i = \frac{1}{N} \sum_{n=1}^{N} \left|x_{o,i}[n]\right|^2 \tag{8.3}$$

8.4 DERIVATION OF THE PROBABILITY OF DETECTION AND THE PROBABILITY OF FALSE ALARM

In essence, the decision variable given in (8.3) can be reformulated in the indefinite quadratic form (IQF):

$$y_i = \frac{1}{N} \| x \|^2 = \| x \|^2_{\frac{1}{N}I} \tag{8.4}$$

Without loss of generality, we assume that

$x = \left[x_{o,i}[1], x_{o,i}[2], x_{o,i}[3], \ldots, x_{o,i}[N] \right]^T$ is complex Gaussian with zero mean and correlation matrix R_x. Where $R_x = E\left[x_i x_i^H \right] = \sigma_x I$, I is the identity matrix for uncorrelated x_i.

Now let $\tilde{x} \sim \mathcal{N}(0, I)$ be the whitened version of $x \sim \mathcal{N}(0, R_x)$

$$\tilde{x} = R_x^{-H/2} x$$

Thus, we rewrite y_i in terms of matrix A as

$$y_i = \| x \|^2_A$$

where

$$A = R_x^{1/2} \frac{1}{N} I R_x^{H/2} = \sigma I_x \frac{1}{N} I \sigma_x I^H = \frac{\sigma_x^2}{N} I = \begin{bmatrix} \dfrac{\sigma_x^2}{N} & 0 & 0 \\ 0 & \dfrac{\sigma_x^2}{N} & 0 \\ 0 & 0 & \dfrac{\sigma_x^2}{N} \end{bmatrix}$$

Here, σ_x^2 is the signal energy depending on the hypothesis H_0 / H_1. Thus, it can be evaluated as

$$\sigma_x^2 = \begin{cases} \displaystyle\sum_{c=1}^{c} E_c T_r \left[R_c w w^H \right] + \sigma_n^2; H_0 \\ E_o T_r \left[R_o w w^H \right] + \displaystyle\sum_{c=1}^{c} E_c T_r \left[R_c w w^H \right] + \sigma_n^2; H_1 \end{cases} \tag{8.5}$$

The probability of detection (p_d) and the probability of false alarm (p_f) for the ith CR relay can be obtained by evaluating the following probabilities:

$$p_{d_i} = p_r\left(y_i > \varepsilon_i | H_1 \right) = 1 - p_r\left(y_i < \varepsilon_i | H_1 \right) \tag{8.6}$$

$$P_{f_i} = p_r\left(y_i > \varepsilon_i|H_0\right) = 1 - p_r\left(y_i < \varepsilon_i|H_0\right) \tag{8.7}$$

The probabilities $p_r\left(y < \varepsilon|H_o\right)$ and $p_r\left(y < \varepsilon|H_1\right)$ can be found similarly as Equation (24) from [24].

$$F_{y_i} = p_r\left(y_i < \varepsilon_i|H_k\right) = \frac{1}{2\pi}\int_{-\infty}^{\infty} \frac{1}{|I + (j\omega + \beta)\Lambda|} \frac{e^{y(j\omega + \beta)}}{(j\omega + \beta)} \delta\omega$$

Since all diagonal elements are the same in a whited matrix A, all eigenvalues are the same, $\lambda = \lambda_1 = \lambda_2 = \dots = \lambda_N = \frac{\sigma_x^2}{N}$. Then to solve the above integration, we need to apply partial fractions for the inner fraction of the below expression, which can be expanded as:

$$F_{y_i} = \frac{1}{2\pi}\int_{-\infty}^{\infty}\left(\frac{A_0}{(j\omega + \beta)} + \sum_{n=1}^{N} \frac{A_n}{\left(I + (j\omega + \beta)\lambda\right)^N} \right) e^{y(j\omega + \beta)}\delta\omega$$

After simplifying the partial fraction, the evaluation of $A_0 = 1, A_n = -\lambda$ which results in the following two integrals:

$$F_{y_i} = \frac{1}{2\pi}\int_{-\infty}^{\infty} \frac{1}{(j\omega + \beta)} e^{y(j\omega + \beta)}\delta\omega + \frac{1}{2\pi}\int_{-\infty}^{\infty}\sum_{n=1}^{N} \frac{-\lambda}{\left(I + (j\omega + \beta)\lambda\right)^n} e^{y(j\omega + \beta)}\delta\omega$$

Hence, applying the residue theory approach of [24], we can formulate the final CDF as below:

$$p_r\left(y_i < \varepsilon_i|H_k\right) = u(y) - \sum_{n=1}^{N} \frac{sign^n(\lambda)}{\lambda^{n-1}\Gamma(n)} y^{n-1} e^{\frac{-y}{\lambda}} u\left(\frac{y}{\lambda}\right) \tag{8.8}$$

for k = 0, 1.

8.5 PROPOSED HEURISTIC METHODS FOR SPECTRUM SENSING OPTIMIZATION

In the proposed solution, we develop heuristic algorithms to obtain the optimum solution for beam vector w by maximizing the probability of detection while constraining the probability of false alarm to some threshold value, that is:

$$\min_{w} J(w) = p_{d_i}(w) \tag{8.9}$$

subject to $p_{f_i} \le \alpha$
where α is some acceptable level of probability of false alarm. To implement the above optimization task, we implement two heuristic algorithms. Namely, the genetic

algorithm with multiparent crossover (GA-MPC) and the cross entropy (CE) optimization methods, which are explained next.

8.5.1 GENETIC ALGORITHM WITH MULTI PARENT CROSSOVER

The genetic algorithm (GA) is a well-known heuristic optimization technique which has been applied to numerous real-world optimization problems. In the GA, there are two main operations involved which are crossover and mutation. There are different techniques to perform these operations. In this context, various multi-parent crossover operations are developed such as simplex crossover, parent centric crossover, triangular crossover, and unimodal distribution crossover. Elsayed et al. [25] proposed a multi-parent crossover operation based on the mutation strategy of differential evolution. The GA-MPC has shown superior performance in contrast to classical single parent crossover based GA. Thus, the GA-MPC has been successfully applied in various well known problems such as static and dynamic dispatching, transmission networks, catalyst blends, benchmark functions planning, transmission pricing, optimal control, and antenna design.

8.5.1.1 GA-MPC Crossover Operation

The process of crossover in the GA-MPC involves five major steps that are as follows:

1. A selection pool is prepared by selecting various chromosomes using the defined selection operation.
2. In order to avoid duplication, the selected parents are checked and the duplicated one is replaced by a random chromosome from the selection pool.
3. The selected parents are sorted w.r.t. to their level of best fit.
4. A tuning parameter β to control the crossover operation is initialized randomly.
5. Finally, the three offspring are generated according to the following equations:

$$\vec{o}_1 = \vec{x}_1 + \left[\beta \times \left(\vec{x}_2 - \vec{x}_3 \right) \right]$$

$$\vec{o}_2 = \vec{x}_2 + \left[\beta \times \left(\vec{x}_3 - \vec{x}_1 \right) \right]$$

$$\vec{o}_3 = \vec{x}_3 + \left[\beta \times \left(\vec{x}_1 - \vec{x}_2 \right) \right]$$

8.5.2 CROSS ENTROPY METHOD

The cross-entropy (CE) method was originally proposed to perform continuous optimization [26] and to estimate rare event probabilities [27]. This method is a Monte Carlo technique [26]. If the CE method is used for an optimization task, the optimization problem is first transformed to rare event estimation problem and then the CE method is employed using cross entropy as a similarity measure between the two variables which can be the target output and the GA-MPC output. The CE method can be implemented via stochastic optimization as explained in [28].

8.5.3 OVERALL IMPLEMENTATION OF THE PROPOSED SCHEME

The GA-MPC and the proposed CE based scheme is presented in [29]. The overall implementation of the proposed scheme involves the following steps:

1. Initialize random population for the GA-MPC.
2. Save the best chromosome for future utilization.
3. Apply tournament selection for the offspring generation.
4. Apply a multi-parent crossover operation using the procedure provided in Section 8.5.1.1.
5. Apply diversity operation for the GA-MPC.
6. Evaluate the objective function or the cost function. If the criterion is met, save the result, otherwise repeat steps (1–5).

8.6 RESULTS AND DISCUSSION

The results provided in this section are obtained from the recently published patent [29]. We consider the average transmitted symbol energy of PU signal and CCI (E_o/E_c) equal to 1. Besides that, the channel fading coefficients $h_{o,i}^H$ and $h_{c,i}^H$ are generated randomly for the PU channel and each CCI channel. Also, the noise variance of the additive white Gaussian (AWG) is considered constant in the channels as ($\sigma_n^2 = 0.01$). The experiment is done for a node that is experiencing several CCI nodes (CCI = 5) which transmit samples (N = 5) and receive the signals via five different antenna elements ($A_M = 5$). The tuning parameters of the GA-MPC and the CE are selected after various trails and are provided in Table 8.2 [29].

TABLE 8.1
Parameter Settings for GA-MPC and CE Algorithms

Parameters	GA-MPC Parameters	CE parameter
Population size	100	100
No. of iteration	100	100
Range of Search Space	{0,1}	{0,1}
Weightings	Complex Random	Complex Random
Probability of Crossover	70%	-
Probability of Diversity	20%	-
Elite Sample (N^{elite})	-	5
Beta (β)	-	98%
Alpha (α)	-	50%
Integer (q)	-	9

Source: [29].

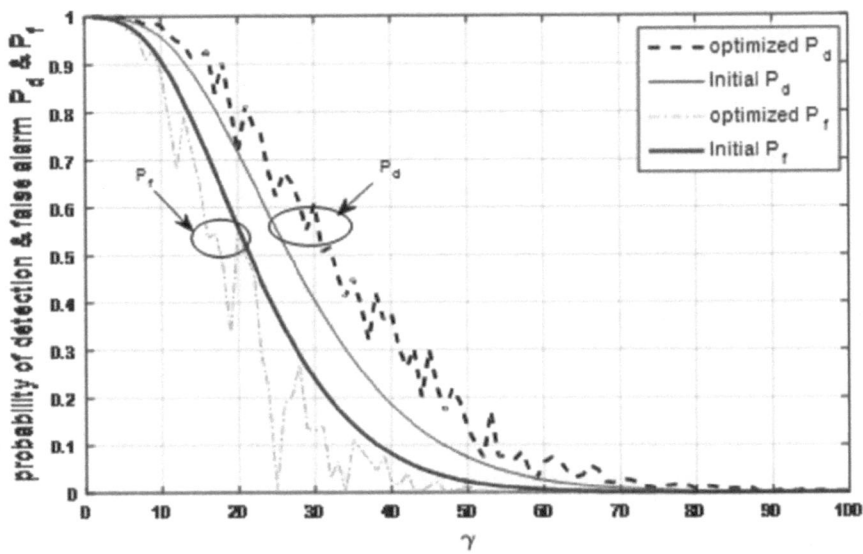

FIGURE 8.4   Optimized p_{d_i} corresponding to its lowest p_{f_i} via the GA_MPC Algorithm [29].

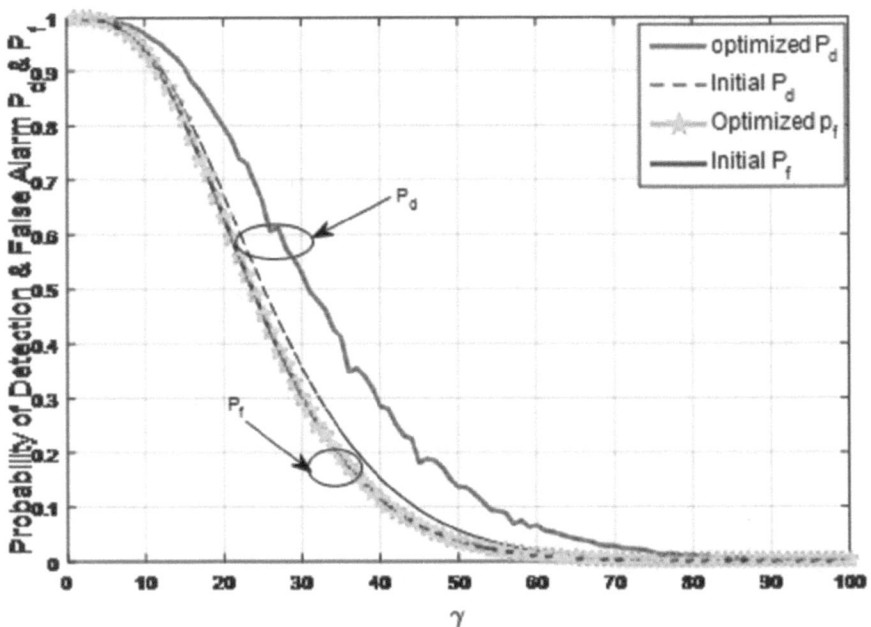

FIGURE 8.5   Optimized p_{d_i} corresponding to its lowest p_{f_i} via the CE Algorithm [29].

Optimized p_d by way of a GA-MPC optimization technique can be seen in Figure 8.4. It has been proven that the GA-MPC was able to optimize this complex problem while considering the lowest level of p_f as clearly shown in the green curve within the same figure. As seen in the same figure, the optimized p_d is improved compared with its Benchmark p_d. Similarly, for p_f which is minimized compared to its corresponding standard p_f.

On the other hand, CE is applied to optimize p_d with respect to the constraint p_f (namely, p_f lower than a certain target). The performance plotted in Figure 8.5 is good, where the optimized p_d shows improvements compared with the standard initial p_d.

8.7 CONCLUSION

In this chapter, we have studied the task of spectrum sensing in the CRN. We considered the ED method of spectrum sensing. For this task, we first derived the probability of detection and the probability of false alarm in closed form using the approach of indefinite quadratic forms. Then, we developed two heuristic methods, GA-MPC and CE, to solve a constrained optimization problem that maximizes the probability of detection while constraining the probability of false alarm to less than a certain acceptable level. The results show that the CE algorithm has better performance than the GA-MPC algorithm.

REFERENCES

1. "Spectrum policy task force report," Federal Communication Commission, Washington, DC, USA, Tech. Rep. 02–155, Nov. 2002.
2. Akyildiz, I. F., Lee, W-Y., Vuran, M. C., and Mohanty, S. "Next generation/dynamic spectrum access/cognitive radio wireless networks: A survey," *Computer Networks*, vol. 50, no. 13, 2006.
3. Haykin, S. "Cognitive radio: brain-empowered wireless communications," *IEEE Journal on Selected Areas in Communications*, vol. 23, no. 2, pp. 201–220, Feb. 2005.
4. Duan, D., Yang, L., and Principe, J. C. "Cooperative diversity of spectrum sensing for cognitive radio systems," *IEEE Trans. Signal Process.*, vol. 58, no. 6, pp. 3218–3227, Jun. 2010.
5. Quan, Z., Cui, S., Sayed, A. H., and Poor, H. V. "Optimal multiband jointdetection forspectrum sensing in cognitive radio networks," *IEEE Trans. Signal Process.*, vol. 57, no. 3, pp. 1128–1140, May 2009.
6. Digham, F., Alouini, M. S., and Simon, M. K. "On the energy detection of unknown signals over fading channels," *IEEE Trans. Commun.*, vol. 55, no. 1, pp. 21–24, Jan. 2007.
7. Atapattu, S., Tellambura, C., and Jiang, H. "Energy-detection-based cooperative spectrum sensing in cognitive radio networks," *IEEE Trans. Wireless Commun.*, vol. 10, no. 4, pp. 1232–1241, Apr. 2011.
8. Zeng, W., and Bi, G. "Exploiting the multipath diversity and multiuser cooperation to detect OFDM signals for cognitive radio in low SNR with noise uncertainty," in *Proc. IEEE Global Telecommun. Conf.*, pp. 1–6, Dec. 2009.

9. Han, W., Li, J., Tian, Z., and Zhang, Y. "Efficient cooperative spectrum sensing with minimum overhead in cognitive radio," *IEEE Trans. Wireless Commun.*, vol. 9, no. 10, pp. 3006–3011, Oct. 2010.

10. Cabric, D., Mishra, S. M., and Brodersen, R.W. "Implementation Issues in Spectrum Sensing for Cognitive Radios," in *Proc. 38th Asilomar Conference on Signals, Systems and Computers*, 2004.

11. Ganesan, G., and Li, Y. "Cooperative spectrum sensing in cognitive radio, Part I: Two user networks," *IEEE Transactions on Wireless Communications*, vol. 6, no. 6, pp. 2204–2213, June 2007.

12. Chair, Z., and Varshney, P.K., "Optimal data fusion in multiple sensor detection systems," *IEEE Trans. on Aerospace and Elect. Syst.*, vol. 22, pp. 98–101, 1986.

13. Visotsky, E., Kuffner, S., and Peterson, R. "On Collaborative Detection of TV Transmissions in Support of Dynamic Spectrum Sharing," *First IEEE International Symposium on New Frontiers in Dynamic Spectrum Access Networks, 2005. DySPAN 2005.*, Baltimore, MD, USA, pp. 338–345, 2005.

14. Digham, F. F., Alouini, M., and Simon, M. K. "On the energy detection of unknown signals over fading channels," *IEEE Transactions on Communications*, vol. 55, no. 1, pp. 21–24, Jan. 2007.

15. Flajolet, P., and Martin, G. N. "Probabilistic counting algorithms for data base applications," *Journal of Computer and System Sciences*, vol. 31, no. 2, pp. 182–209, Oct. 1985.

16. Niu, R., and Varshney, P. K. "Distributed detection and fusion in a large wireless sensor network of random size," *EURASIP Journal onWireless Communications and Networking*, vol. 815873, pp. 462–472, 2005, https://doi.org/10.1155/WCN.2005.462.

17. Zhang, W., Mallik, R. K., and Letaief, K. B. "Cooperative Spectrum Sensing Optimization in Cognitive Radio Networks," *2008 IEEE International Conference on Communications*, Beijing, pp. 3411–3415, 2008.

18. Ma, J., and Li, Y. G. "Soft Combination and Detection for Cooperative Spectrum Sensing in Cognitive Radio Networks," *IEEE GLOBECOM 2007–IEEE Global Telecommunications Conference*, Washington, DC, pp. 3139–3143, 2007.

19. El-Saleh, A., Ismail, M., Ali, M., and Al-kebsi, "Capacity Enhancement and Interference Reduction in Cooperative Cognitive Radio Networks," *Future Computer and Communication (ICFCC), International Conference, Kuala Lumpur, Malaysia*, 2009.

20. Liang, Y., Zeng, Y., Peh, E. C. Y., and Hoang, A. T. "Sensing-throughput tradeoff for cognitive radio networks," *IEEE Transactions on Wireless Communications*, vol. 7, no. 4, pp. 1326–1337, April 2008.

21. Peh, E., and Liang, Y-C. "Optimization for Cooperative Sensing in Cognitive Radio Networks," *Wireless Communications and Networking Conference*, IEEE, March 2007.

22. Shen, B., Huang, L., Zhao, C., Kwak, K., and Zhou, Z. "Weighted Cooperative Spectrum Sensing in Cognitive Radio Networks," *2008 Third International Conference on Convergence and Hybrid Information Technology*, Busan, pp. 1074–1079, 2008.

23. Lehtomaki, J., Juntti, M., Saarnisaari, H., and Koivu, S. "Threshold setting strategies for a quantized total power radiometer," *IEEE SignalProcessing Lett.*, vol. 12, no. 11, pp. 796–799, Nov. 2005.

24. T. Y. Al-Naffouri, M. Moinuddin, N. Ajeeb, B. Hassibi, and A. L. Moustakas, "On the distribution of indefinite quadratic forms in Gaussian random variables," *IEEE Transactions on Communications*, vol. 64, pp. 153–165, 2016.

25. Elsayed, S. M., Sarker, R. A., and Essam, D. L. "A new genetic algorithm for solving optimization problems," *Engineering Applications of Artificial Intelligence*, vol. 27, pp. 57–69, Jan. 2014.

26. Rubinstein, R. Y. The cross-entropy method for combinatorial and continuous optimization. *Methodologyand Computing in Applied Probability*, vol. 1, no.2, pp. 127–190, 1999.

27. Rubinstein, R. Y. Combinatorial optimization, cross-entropy, ants and rare events. In S. Uryasev and P. M. Pardalos (Eds.), *Stochastic Optimization: Algorithmsand Applications* (pp. 304–358). Dordrecht: Kluwer, 2001.

28. Rubinstein, R., and Kroese, D. P. *The Cross-Entropy Method: A Unified Approach to Combinatorial Optimization, Monte-Carlo Simulation and Machine Learning.* Springer-Verlag, 2004.

29. Moinuddin, M., Al-Saggaf, U. M., Alrefaei, M. A., and Ahmad, J. "Communications device with antenna-based spectrum sensing without gaussian assumption", US Patent US11218885B2, Jan. 2022.

9 Gamified Wearables in Childhood Obesity Therapy Driven by 5G Wireless Communication System with Special Emphasis on Pacific Island Countries

Pragya Singh

CONTENTS

DOI: 10.1201/9781003368311-9

9.1 INTRODUCTION

In current years, gaining weight, being overweight and being obese have become social problems. It is classified as a chronic condition by both the American Medical Association (AMA) and the World Health Organization (WHO) [1]. Obesity can lead to other chronic diseases such as diabetes and cardiovascular disease, which are important causes of death and disability around the world. Obesity is an economic liability on health systems especially in the case of developing countries. This leads to impaired educational and cognitive development in children [2]. Reports from the National Institute of Health and Nutrition have shown that the global obesity epidemic has progressively expanded since 1970, with the prevalence of obesity having more than tripled, particularly among children and adolescents [3]. As a result, childhood obesity may be regarded as one of the most pressing public health concerns in the twenty-first century. Florence et al. have reported that this is the reason that explains 27% of the increase in medical costs between 1987 and 2001 [4]. According to the World Health Organization, there will be 70 million overweight or obese children in the world by 2025 [5]. Obese children usually have high chances of dying prematurely and of suffering from NCDs that may lead to adulthood disability and have serious effects on mental health so there is an urgent need to design an effective intervention strategy that can help children, adolescents, and obese adults [6]. Despite the fact that various intervention strategies have been tested, the incidence of obesity in children and adolescents continues to rise. The issue that remains is, how can current programs for obesity prevention be made more effective? So, the present study is undertaken with the objective to gain insight into how gamification is being applied to obesity prevention and treatment in children and adolescents. To study which game designs were used and tested on the target audience and how effective the use of gamification was in the prevention of obesity and the development of the practice of healthy eating and physical activity in children and adolescents.

A rigorous literature search was conducted, based on five stages of grounded theory using the method of Wolfswinkel et al. [7]. Before the first search of the database, a variety of probable search terms were determined to confirm the relevance of the topic to science. The main search terms used included: obese/overweight children, childhood/adolescence obesity, weight loss, health applications, physical activity, serious games, gamification, wearable devices, and smartphones. These terms are sufficient to describe the problem and reflect the scope of the roles of 5G in gamified wearables for childhood obesity.

Thanks to the original speed improvements, 5G can offer amazing speeds up to 10 Gbps, 10 times the speed of video gamers compared to 4G LTE. Children and adolescents can all expect faster downloads and streaming, and the delays in downloading and streamlining have been significantly improved. Response times are as short as 5 mins, making in-game actions smoother than ever and eliminating lag between input and game response. This is true even if a large number of simultaneous players are using a mobile application, due to the high reliability of 5G.

The original speed of 5G isn't only about the advantages it provides to gaming. Higher bandwidth and shorter response times mean that cloud computing will be more feasible. This enables developers to tackle more demanding and complex jobs from afar and deliver higher-quality results to players. This reduces people's worries about whether the game will run on older or lower spec phones. End users can play higher-quality games as long as they have a 5G data subscription. 5G technological advances will drive the next wave of mobile innovation, especially in the field of mobile gaming. With exponential download and upload speeds, anyone can download mobile games almost instantly. Large mobile games (over 100 MB) can be downloaded at once without the hassle of downloading other content in the first release, so players can get the content immediately. Nintendo's mobile RPG game "Dragalia Lost" is a good example of this annoyance, as the player has to download other content first and then download new levels as he progresses.

Due to the inevitability of cell phones, IoT-based wearable gadgets, and personal computers, gamification has garnered a lot of attention recently in the medical care profession [8]. A new study from the Pennington Center for Biomedical Research at Louisiana State University showed that by integrating video games with fitness trainers and footstep trackers, overweight children can lose weight, decrease blood pressure and cholesterol, and boost physical activity.

Children who gain too much weight without exercising have early warning symptoms of heart disease and diabetes. Dr. Amanda Steiano, director of the Institute for Childhood Obesity and Health Behavior at Pennington Biomedical and a principal investigator in the study explained that in Louisiana, one-third (35.3%) of children aged 10 to 17 are overweight or obese, and one-fifth (21.1%) suffer from obesity, according to data from the US Centers for Disease Control and Prevention. All people face an increased risk of developing serious medical problems due to obesity. It may be helpful to play a video game that requires exercise. Dr. Steiano said: "Screens are everywhere in our lives. Children wake up and spend half of their time in front of small screens. I'm searching for procedures to use these screens, smartphones, laptops, computers, TV, tablets to integrate more sporting activities into children's lives.

9.2   DEFINING OBESITY

Obesity is described by the World Health Organization (WHO) as "an increase in excessive body fat that probably influence and impair health" [9, 10]. BMI, which is defined as a person's weight in kilograms divided by the square of their height in meters (kg/m²), is used to define overweight and obesity. According to the WHO, an adult with a BMI of more than 25 kg/m² is overweight, while one with a BMI of more than or equal to 30 kg/m² is obese. These standard BMI cut-off values for adults are now generally utilized for all genders, regardless of age [9].

Obesity in children is described as an excess of adipose tissue that affects the health and well-being of the child. Defining overweight and obese using BMI for age may be differently used between countries as it depends on the reference data and cut-offs used [11]. According to the WHO cut-offs, a child or adolescent is overweight if his/her BMI for age and sex is > 1 SD and obese if BMI is >2 SD above the average or median [12]. The Centre for Disease Control and Prevention (CDC) cut-offs define overweight as ≥ 85th but < 95th percentiles, and ≥ 95th percentile as obese as per age-specific BMI charts developed by the CDC [13].

9.3   GLOBAL TRENDS AMONG CHILDREN

Childhood obesity is on the rise around the world, with disturbing trends in the United States, United Kingdom, and other wealthy countries, as well as in low- and middle-income countries [14]. CPOND [15] published a report in 2015 on situational analysis of child BMI monitoring in the Pacific Islands and Territories (PICTS) Information on prevalence and trends in childhood obesity is missing in many PICTs. Likewise, there is inadequate information on existing systems for regular childhood BMI monitoring in a minimum of 16 Pacific Island countries. The Children's Healthy Living (CHL) Project [16], in collaboration with government agencies initiatives, and communities throughout the northern United States affiliated Pacific Islands (USAPI) region, had developed a child BMI monitoring approach. The CHL program stresses American Samoa, the Commonwealth of the Northern Marianas (CNMI), the Freely Associated States of Micronesia (Republic of Marshall Islands, Palau, FSM), Guam, and Hawaii. The goal of the initiative was to address childhood obesity through various environments (social/cultural, political/economic, physical, and built). The key component of the program is to establish a standardized monitoring system for child BMI.

In partnership with Head Start (Early Childhood Agencies) and the US government program for early childhood education (ECE), the project targets BMI monitoring of 2–8 years old children in pre-schools. Measurements of BMI of children 5–8 years is conducted twice a year (starting and finishing the school year) by teachers in ECE and is compulsory. CHL has been involved in the standardization of anthropometric measures through the training of trainers and the development of standardization protocols and courses [17]. Of the 16 PICTs, four countries have an established system of periodic BMI measurements in children which are Fiji, the Cook Islands, New Caledonia, and French Polynesia. Tuvalu also reported conducting a survey of childhood BMI in selected primary schools, with childhood BMI measurements done on an ad-hoc basis. The prevalence of overweight was 19.6% while obesity was 16.2% in the survey conducted by the Health Directorate in French Polynesia in 2014 in the age group of 7–9 years. The Sanitary and Social agency of New Caledonia (ASSNC) conducted a cross-sectional survey in 2012 among children aged 6, 9 and 12 years old in New Caledonia and found out the prevalence of obesity as 7.8%, 11.4% and 20.5 % respectively.

According to several research projects, the prevalence of overweight and obesity in children and adolescents in Fiji varies. One study reported overweight in Fijian adolescents between the ages of 12–14 at 15.2% and 15–18 year olds at 17.4%. When categorized according to ethnicity, 24.9% of I-Taukei adolescents between the ages of 12–18 years were overweight and 9.8% of Fijians of Indian-descent were overweight [18]. The Global Burden of Disease study in 2013 estimated a prevalence of overweight and obesity as 12.8 % among boys (less than 20 years of age) and 24.9% among girls in a similar age group in the Fiji Islands [19]. The rate of overweight and obesity increased from 4.7% to 7.2% in children between the ages of 5 and 14 years from the National Nutritional Survey (NNS) 2004 to the National Nutrition Survey (NNS) 2016 while the rate of overweight and obesity increased from 6.2% to 8.1% in adolescents 15 to 17 years of age from NNS 2004 to NNS 2016 [20]. Figures 9.1 and 9.2 illustrate the distribution of obesity among different ethnic groups in Fiji [20].

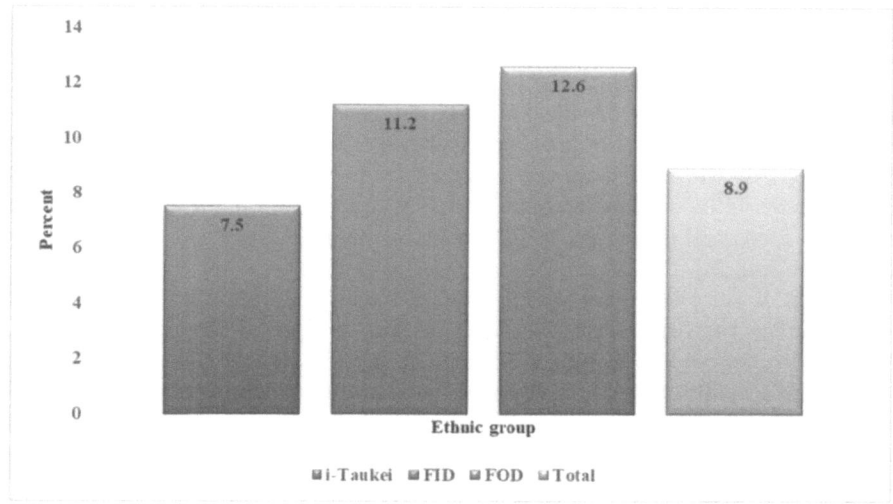

FIGURE 9.1   Distribution of overweight and obesity in children (5–14 years old) across various ethnic groups in Fiji [20].

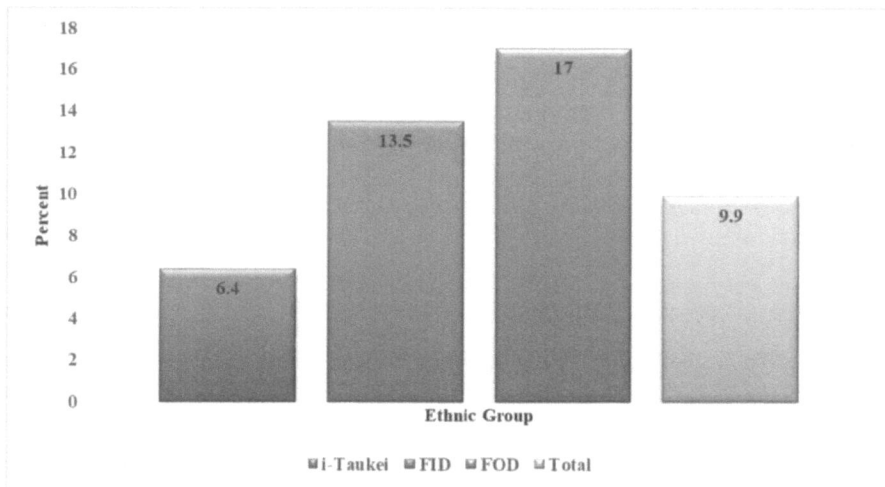

FIGURE 9.2   Distribution of overweight and obesity in adolescents (15–17 years old) across different ethnic group in Fiji [20].

9.4   RISK FACTORS FOR CHILDHOOD OBESITY

Overweight and obesity result from the interaction of genetic, physiological, environmental, and psychological factors which results in a chronic imbalance between energy consumption (from foods and drinks) and energy expenditure (physical activity). Davison and Birch suggest that the following are risk factors for childhood obesity: dietary intake, physical inactivity, and sedentary behavior [21]. Environmental and behavioral changes over the past few decades have led to the prevalence of rising rates of obesity. Children grow up in a "obesogenic environment," where unhealthy foods are more readily available, inexpensive, and enticing [22]. Fast foods with their ease and convenience have replaced home-made meals and the media influences the eating choices of children through the advertising of unhealthy foods and beverages. It is also known that portion size control protects against obesity [23].

Physical activity has been greatly reduced with the children spending more time on screen-based activities [24]. With the ease and speed of modern transport, walking to school is less common. Schools, in particular, have a special influence on children's health with their physical education curriculum and school-based canteens providing lunch and snacks for students. Parental factors also have an impact on obesity with their behavior, attitudes and feeding styles mimicked by their children [25].

9.5   EFFECTS OF CHILDHOOD OBESITY

9.5.1   Medical Effects

Medical conditions that have been more prevalent among adolescents include type 2 diabetes, fatty liver, orthopedic problems, and sleep apnea [26]. Obesity is also harmful to the cardiovascular system and being overweight during childhood exacerbates and accelerates cardiovascular conditions in adulthood. The fact that life expectancy is decreasing could be attributed to children developing obesity at a younger age and thus developing various non-communicable diseases earlier and ultimately premature death [27, 28]. In fact, studies have reported a near doubling of hospitalizations due to childhood obesity [29].

9.5.2   Social and Academic Effects

A study evaluated the health-related quality of life of obese and non-obese children and discovered that obese children were more likely to have decreased health-related quality of life, including emotional, social, and school functioning, as compared to healthy children [30]. Further studies on self-esteem in the United States showed significantly poorer levels of self-esteem in early adolescents in obese Hispanic and white females and showed higher rates of sadness and nervousness and adolescents being more prone to participation in risky habits such as smoking or consuming alcohol [31]. This in turn would affect academic performance in otherwise normal, healthy children. Moreover, obesity that continues further to adulthood is associated with poorer employment and relationship outcomes [32]. The effects of both medical and social effects of obesity in children have not been studied in detail in the South Pacific (Figure 9.3).

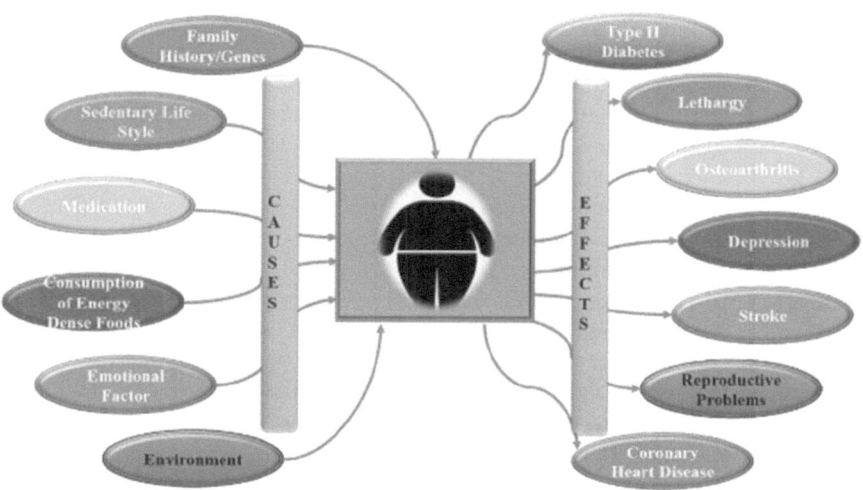

FIGURE 9.3 Diagrammatic representation of the causes and effects of childhood obesity.

9.6 SELF-DETERMINATION THEORY (SDT) AND OBESITY PREVENTION

All modern lifestyle risk factors are directly affected by the person's health behavior, whether it be related to diet, physical activity, screen-based behaviors, sleep time, and the like. According to self-determination theory (SDT), not all forms of motivation have an equal effect on behaviors. An important consideration is whether the behavior is intrinsically or extrinsically motivated. Intrinsically motivated behavior constitutes that behavior for which an individual performs activities in order to meet their own purposes which fulfil the basic physiological needs for autonomy, competence, and relatedness, resulting in a feeling of willingness and pleasure. Extrinsically motivated behavior is done due to external demand or reward. Such behaviors have an external line of control [33]. In the present times, STD has become a vital framework for designing interventions in the field of health care. Various studies have shown a positive impact of using intrinsic motivation over extrinsic motivation which leads to sustainable desired behavioral change. A person's health and wellbeing are related to a person's health behaviors and motivation is an important factor for health behavior change and intrinsically motivated behavior change is sustainable and contributes to the health and wellbeing of an individual [34]. This leads to the very important question of what type of intervention will bring about a sustainable health behavior change. Positive computing [35] or persuasive technology [36] can provide an answer to this question. Positive computing is often used to focus people's attention on particular facts that can bring about a change in their thinking and behaviors. It is a computer system, mobile application, device, and so forth, that is intentionally designed to bring about a change in a user's behavior and action. This includes tools or wearables (for example, pedometers), media (audio, video, or both) and social interactive games (playing with another person) to assist the person to alter their behavior [37]. The important sector in this category is games for health. These are the games designed to achieve health-related outcomes. In this category, most popular are the games targeting physical activity, nutrition, stroke rehabilitation. Like all other games, these games have also witnessed an increased growth in the last two decades. Positive computing is playing a vital part in the prevention of overweight and obesity. It is mostly used by kids in the age range of 12 to 17 years. Some examples include game consoles and Nintendo Wii games. The subjects who use these attain certain skills which can be used in other activities which lead to physical, social, and cognitive development. In these games, the subject becomes the creator of the contents when the character movements are controlled by the uses of the subject's body actions. Exergames imitate the physical movement of the subject and store it as input associated to the specific meaning of gameplay. This is then transformed into three-dimensional movements on a two-dimensional screen. This helps to improve visual-spatial abilities, hand-eye, and foot-eye coordination in the subject. It also helps to improve his virtual and social interaction as the subject competes in a time within a given period [36]. The major disadvantage is that the subject requires a dedicated device, space, and time for the gameplay. The cost incurred in the design and production is also high and the development of such games is a time-intensive process.

9.7 GAMIFICATION

Gamification is one major field of research which has gained a lot of attention for use in many sectors such as education, health care, human resources, cooperate management to promote sports throughout the world due to increased use of smartphones, laptops, and computers. Although Pacific Island countries are seeing moderate growth in mobile users of just 30% of connections at the end of 2018, this is forecast to more than double to 65% by 2025 [38]. Gamification is a creative way of motivating people and encouraging change in them through the use of game features that are aimed to engage the subject in a non-game context. Game elements stimulate a feeling of happiness and hence ultimately enrich the skill of users [39]. Sailer et al. [40] listed the most fundamental game design features used within a gamification setting as follows:

- Points: Prizes collected for certain activities
- Badges: Pictorial signs of successes, which can be collected in the gaming environment
- Leaderboards: Providing information about performer's successes, based on points or badges which a performer has earned, with all the performers are ranked on leaderboards
- Progress bars: Statistics about a performer's existing position towards accomplishing an aim
- Performance graphs: Giving evidence about a performer's performance in the game that the player is currently playing against his performances in previous attempts
- Avatars: Graphical images of the performers.

Gamification design involves using the above-mentioned tools to impact inspirational efficiency and players' actions in a positive manner. Only a few research projects have been conducted to assess the psychological consequences of gamification as well as its impacts on behavioral change. However, Sailer et al. [40] attempted to study the association of gamification to six principal perspectives of motivational research. According to HAPA, motivation can be perceived as a step that results in the development of a target behavior, afterwards developing the desire in the subject to follow that behavior. In the motivational phase, people become inspired to modify their behavior when addressing features such as social guidance, awareness including customs and modeling, and self-efficacy anticipations. Several researchers have claimed that gamification can decrease the internal motivation for an activity performed by a user as in this case the user starts acting under external motivation and not under internal motivation [41]. Others suggest that extrinsic motivation prizes, attained through competitive aims, can be viewed as an effective tool while intrinsic motivation is still growing [33]. If the user can realize the significance of the information provided by gamification design, then intrinsic motivation can be enhanced as there is less requirement to stress the importance of external reward. However, when aiming at "intenders" the combination of external motivation employing instantaneous response, by use of points conferred for positive actions and the picturing of growth using a progress bar, could assist to motivate behavior or reimburse for the absence of intrinsic motivation in the direction of long-term change in nutritional behavior. A leaderboard function would let users to relate themselves to other players in a reference group (for example, their close peers) in real time, allowing them to evaluate their strengths and encouraging healthy competition.

A sense of achievement may emerge for "intenders" at the top of a leaderboard, along with emotions of social affinity due to common goals and involvements, leading to an improved sense of self-efficacy and intrinsic motivation [42]. At the same time, the leaderboard represents a descriptive social model by supplying evidence on the "normal" behavior of significant others. This is especially significant for insecure persons who are uncertain if they will be able to change because they may be striving to continue since complying with the observed social standard and obtaining feedback would let them determine how close they are to the established standard. This would be considerably more successful if they were close to the other players involved (proximal reference group). As "intenders" are inspired to make changes but are hampered by feelings of insecurity, this lack of self-efficacy could be alleviated. Gamification, if properly planned and implemented, has the potential to kick-start a process that promotes behavioral changes. It may work as an intervention affecting social norms and self-efficacy by providing knowledge about reference group norms relative to the behavior of oneself and important others.

9.7.1 ADVANTAGES OF GAMIFICATION FOR USE IN HEALTH AND WELLBEING

The reason why the use of gamification is more suitable for health and behavior change today is due to shortcomings in other types of interventions that are as follows:

1. Intrinsic motivation: Gamified systems intrinsically motivate and continue the performance of the activities which lead to health and wellbeing [43–45] in comparison to other intervention techniques where extrinsic motivation such as social pressure or where overt rewards are used because of which these interventions lacked sustainable appeal [46].
2. Broad appeal: The use of mobile game applications is increasing in all of the audiences, ranging from children as small as 3 years old to the elderly [44]. On this basis, health messages around healthy eating practices regarding childhood obesity which involves children, their caretakers and health workers can be efficiently delivered to three different types of target audience using a single mobile application, by using different modules.
3. Extensive reach through mobile technology and omnipresent sensors: The activity tracker and smartphone are equipped with sophisticated sensing, processing, storage, and display capabilities, are excellent and widely available platforms for expanding the game layer on a daily basis. So it is advantageous to use these for the delivery of health messages as it does not require any additional external devices [44], [47].
4. Wide range of applicability: Recent health-related gamification includes all key health topics that can cause risks to the population such as physical activity, diet management, weight management, medication adherence, mental wellbeing, and so forth [33].
5. Everyday life fit: These gamified systems using smartphones and trackers can practically track the activities of their users, unlike other health interventions, especially obesity-related interventions, which require dedicated time and space for their execution [43], [33].
6. Cost-effective: These mobile games applications use smartphones which are widely used by different customers and just require the download of the applications, unlike many other interventions which need the use of additional equipment or the dedicated spaces to carry out interventions which incur additional cost to the end users [33].

9.8 WEARABLES

"The terms "wearable technology", "wearable devices", and "wearables" all refer to electronic technologies or tools such as computers that are amalgamated into items of outfit and accessories which can be easily worn on the body." [42], [48]. Wearables occur in numerous devices such as smartwatches, smart glasses, bracelets, gesture controllers or belts [49]. The most common examples are the Apple Watch, the Fitbit bracelet, the controller belt, and Google glasses [50]. The global smart wearables market is anticipated to rise from $13.2 billion in 2019 to $16.12 billion in 2020 at a compound annual growth rate (CAGR) of 22.37% [51]. There has been an increase in the adoption of such wearables as society has recently begun to lean towards a healthier lifestyle [17]. Wearable devices for healthcare and fitness can be classified as technology gadgets and activity trackers that are worn to watch and record a person's physical fitness activity. Wearables are most commonly used for step counting, speed and distance tracking, heart rate tracking, and sleep quality. Bluetooth or Wi-Fi is used to transfer the information to other devices. Despite the fact that wearables can perform many of the core tasks of mobile phones and computers, Tehrani and Michael showed in their publication that the emphasis of wearables is on the provision of sensory, monitoring, and scanning features for health-related data that are normally not present in smartphones and computers, giving them an advantage in this space [52].

9.9 LIMITATIONS OF TECHNOLOGY-BASED INTERVENTIONS

Technology-based interventions have many benefits over traditional in-person models but there are also certain drawbacks. All of the above technology-based interventions require the use of high-speed internet, and the use of smartphones or mobile devices. Internet access varies among different regions of the world especially in island countries where some places have either unstable or no internet connectivity at all. Rural and urban locations, as well as wealthy and impoverished communities, have different levels of connectivity. Furthermore, adopting these technology-based interventions necessitates a certain level of computer or electronic device literacy. Short-term usage of these devices for obesity prevention and weight loss programs has also been found to be promising, but long-term usage has shown mixed results [53].

9.10 BRIEFS FOR INTERVENTION PROGRAMS THAT HAVE USED GAMIFICATION OR WEARABLES IN THE PREVENTION AND CONTROL OF ADOLESCENT AND CHILDHOOD OBESITY

This section describes examples of only those peer-reviewed studies that investigated the effectiveness of gamification on either fruit and vegetable intake or physical activity or both and the research methodologies are clearly explained. Generally, the use of mobile applications, wearables, websites, and the like, is for improving physical activity in adolescence, mental wellbeing in adults and drug adherence in adults. The main studies that are summarized here are those which are either on adolescents or on children to prevent or control obesity in these age groups. Literature has shown that among children and teenagers, using thoughtful games for providing nutritional education can be effective [54, 55]. Numerous studies have looked at the impact of video games on children's and teens' nutritional knowledge and on dietary modification among children and adolescents [56–58]. Schools are generally used as settings for educational (for example, game-based) interventions as a large number of children and adolescents can be found in one place. Additionally, a digital game might be an enjoyable substitute for old-style classroom teaching [54]. Numerous systematic reviews have shown that school-based interventions (for example, fruit and vegetable delivery, water consumption, and physical activity in the form of various sports) can positively impact diet-related outcomes among children and adolescents [59, 60].

The mobile approach to challenge obesity (MACO) developed by Almomani et al., [37] is a game-based persuasive mobile technology, designed to help obese children by providing knowledge about healthy eating and physical activity. The target population for its use was children between the ages of 6 and 12 years. This includes two different types of games. The first is a healthy food game in which the child needs to collect ten healthy foods from all of the foods which drop from the top of the screen before they reach the bottom. The child can only go to the next level once he correctly collects the healthy foods. The second is a physical activity game. In this, there are various types of physical activities such as running, jumping with a certain time allocated for completing each physical activity. Once the activities are finished the user is asked to update the information. The activities are designed in such a way that children will only gain points once they complete their desired activities for a certain period. The child can only move to the next level once they achieve the physical activity time of 60 min and 10 points. 93% of the total children who used MACO agreed that it was enjoyable and 75% agreed that MACO can help them lose weight as if they know healthy and unhealthy foods and do physical activity.

Ezezika et al. had conducted an intervention study in three secondary schools in Abuja, Nigeria for a period of 4 months on understanding the use of gamification to address the problem of unhealthy eating in adolescence (13–17 years old). Nutritional gamification was introduced through board games, clubs, and vouchers. Subjects were asked about their opinions on the intervention and its impact on their knowledge about nutrition, attitudes and eating behavior using focus group discussions. The findings of the focus groups imply that gamification of nutrition can enhance dietary behavior in research participants over the short-term period [61].

Holzmann et al. [62] conducted a preliminary study to assess the immediate efficacy of the "Fit, Food, Fun" (FFF) game, to provide nutritional awareness to children and adolescents in two secondary schools in Bavaria, Germany. The FFF game was created as a voyage across Europe, with each country focusing on food products unique to that region. Three mini games are included in each country. The first game was formulated like a quiz that compares protein, fat, carbohydrates, or calories between two food substances. The second game is planned as an assessment game for the amount of sugar, fat, or salt in one given food substance. The third game can be considered as a physical activity component. Extra points are given for collecting a minimum of five apples during the physical activity component. The next country to visit is revealed after the player completes all three mini-games within one country. The schools were divided into two groups: game play group (GG) and instructional intervention group (TG). The GG intervention consisted of a 15-minute FFF gameplay session every day for three days, while the TG intervention took the form of a regular lecture. Questionnaires were used at baseline and post-intervention to evaluate nutritional knowledge. The results of this study demonstrated that both short-term educational therapies improved children's and adolescent's nutritional understanding, with the TG making more improvement than the GG. Since nutritional knowledge may be lacking in this age group and young people frequently engage in digital gaming, a serious game may be a suitable means of delivering nutritional knowledge in an entertaining setting, but it is still unknown whether the imparted nutritional knowledge can be translated into dietary behavior.

Wang and his colleagues had conducted a study to find out the effect of playing a health video game embedded with story immersion, "Escape from Diab" (Diab), on children's diet and physical activity (PA) and to find out whether children immersed in Diab had better positive outcomes in Chinese children aged 8 to 12 years. Three outcome assessments were done. The first was at baseline, the second soon after the game, and the third after 8–10 weeks when the treatment group played Diab. Children who played Diab had improved intrinsic motivation for fruit and water, self-efficacy for PA, and self-reported PA scores soon after the children played Diab. However, these changes were not significant at 8–10 weeks after playing Diab. Diab provides a promising innovative medium for promoting Chinese children's psychological correlates of diet and PA behavior. Nevertheless, its effectiveness needs to be enhanced and mechanisms of change need to be examined more exhaustively [63].

Del-Rio et al. [64] developed the PROVITAO project, which was an intervention program aimed at promoting healthy habits in obese children aged 6 to 12 years. The research was conducted over the course of three years and was quasi-experimental, longitudinal, and prospective in design. Two different settings were used. The first was children attending HUC's pediatric outpatient clinics (Spain) where the study was conducted in its first year and the second was in public schools of the District of La Laguna, Tenerife, Spain where the study was conducted in its second year. It was divided into two phases, each containing a control and an experimental group in each setting. The PROVITAO project is an important example of the quantified self (QS) proposal. QS is increasingly being used for healthcare with new methods and biometric data analysis. The QS application has many advantages: self-healing, self-discipline, self-improvement, self-knowledge, and so forth. Using this technique, both the healthcare provider and their subject can update information on a measure such as anthropometric data, socioeconomic data, activity data, personal characteristics, diet data, blood test, medical reports, and the like, and this data can be collected and monitored. This is achieved through the use of wearables, mobile phones, apps, activity logs, and exploration. In the first phase the information collected by the medical practitioners in the hospital was given to the research team along with the information relating to the technology network used at home and collected by caregivers. In the second phase, physical education teachers in the participating schools were asked to record information regarding age, weight, height, and sex. There have been serious games and applications developed for educational intervention to promote healthy living. Low-cost heart rate monitors and accelerometers were used to collect the data throughout the study. The PROVITAO app for smartphones and tablets, as well as a portal to gamify the activities accomplished by the children, was developed, and utilized for intervention, with weekly tasks that earned points, rewards, and so on. The results showed no significant improvement in physical activity between the control and experimental group but there was a significant increase related to the knowledge about healthy eating after using it for the long term. The intervention had a positive impact on the emotional development of the children. The application also collected and monitored important participant data throughout the study.

Lee and Gao [65] looked at the impact of iPad and mobile app-based physical education on children's physical activity and psychosocial beliefs. They used 157 fourth and fifth-grade primary school children in two elementary schools in the Midwestern U.S. Children were divided into two groups. The first experimental group served as an app integrated group and the second control group used the traditional PE approach. Three PE sessions were measured for both schools. There was a significant decrease in moderate to vigorous physical activity in the experimental group as compared to the control group. An increase in sedentary time was also observed in the experimental group. The children's psychosocial beliefs were improved in the experimental group as compared to the control group, but the change was not significant. The results may be attributed to the short-term app integration. The teachers were advised to align the use of the app with the goals of PE sessions. The app needs to be carefully selected to increase moderate to vigorous physical activity in the children rather than helping teachers in the management and delivery of their classes.

9.10.1 OBESITY PREVENTION STUDIES CONDUCTED IN PACIFIC ISLAND AND TERRITORIES (PICTS) BY USING GAMIFICATION OR WEARABLES

There are very few studies that have used mobile applications or wearables for preventing or treating obesity in PICTS.

OL@-OR@ mobile phone app and website project [66] was developed and evaluated as a culturally tailored, personalized mobile-phone delivered (mHealth) healthy lifestyle support program for Māori and Pacific Islanders in New Zealand. Users might set goals and invite their whanau and friends to join them in their quest to make healthy lifestyle changes. It includes tools to encourage healthy eating and physical activity, as well as encouraging messages and suggestions on a regular basis. The program was evaluated by a cluster-randomized controlled trial. 337 Māori participants from 19 clusters and 389 Pacific Islander participants from 18 clusters (n = 726 participants) in the intervention group and 320 Māori participants from 15 clusters and 405 Pacific Islander participants from 17 clusters (n = 725 participants) in the control group were the part of the trial. The intervention was conducted for 12 weeks. The main outcome was a 12-week self-reported composite health behavior score that included smoking, vegetable and fruit consumption, alcohol use, and physical activity. The study showed no significant change in health-related behavior in Māori and Pacific Islanders. The OL@-OR@ mobile phone app and website were for adults and not for children or adolescents.

The LAUNCH Legends initiative which is part of the LAUNCH Food platform has developed two pilot projects to determine the possibility of immersive storytelling for the consumption of healthy eating and traditional meals through play-based teaching. Our Special Island for Tonga, and Beyond the Stars was launched for Fiji in 2018. While technology is core to the projects, the Tonga and Fiji initiatives both comprised of the use of an app and the Fiji program also used virtual reality storytelling as the focus, along with flashcards, activity books, and storybooks. Our Special Island was pilot tested in Tonga for six weeks and Beyond the Stars was piloted in Fiji for around ten weeks. The main aim of the pilot testing was to find out how engaging the materials were and not if kids had changed their diets [67].

Galy et al. [68] conducted a pilot intervention study by using digital educational application along with Misfit activity trackers in adolescents 12 to 14 years of age in New Caledonia for 4 weeks. The study aimed to find out the effect of using the educational application program that combines health education, independent measures of physical activity (PA), and self-assessment of aim accomplishment would help the adolescents to achieve the recommended levels of PA. The iEngage program targeted health education, PA-related skills and nutrition guidelines focusing on the sugar content of the foods and the recommended level of sugar consumption. The application consisted of 8 modules each of which was of one hour's duration. Each module consisted of learning activities, quizzes, and short two to five minute PA sessions that generally focused on a specific series of body movements: sprints, jumping, running, walking, squats, or push-ups. The PA was captured by the Misfit activity tracker and sent to the child via the Misfit app through the iEngage modules to maintain learning and offer help in self-assessing accomplishment against personal goals. At the end of each module, the players were guided to set up their aim for the next module. At the end of each module, the player needed to assess if he had achieved the aim which he set at the start of the module. The players were assigned to groups consisting of five players each. The group scored the points if all the members achieved their set goals in their respective modules. The results showed an overall increase of PA during the program, mainly in the less active adolescents who increased their daily steps and there was better adherence to the recommended levels of PA.

Veatupu and his colleagues had conducted a study in Tonga called Me'akai in Tonga by using wearable cameras. These wearable kids' cameras were worn around the neck by randomly selected children between the ages of 10 to 12 years. The study used kids' cameras to study the nature and context of the Me'akai (food) eaten by Tongan children with the help of the pictures taken by the children during three consecutive days when they were wearing these cameras (autographer). The photos taken by these wearable cameras helped to provide a large amount of information regarding the food consumed by these children, for example, the number of meals and snacks consumed by the children, the composition of the meals, food types, the portion sizes of the food consumed, sources of the food, settings where the food was consumed, and how the food was procured (whether purchased or not). The results of this study support the efforts made by the Government of Tonga for the enforcement of a Healthy School Food Policy, junk food taxes, and initiatives to ban the importation of energy-dense nutrient-poor foods in the country [69]. For PICTs it is best to

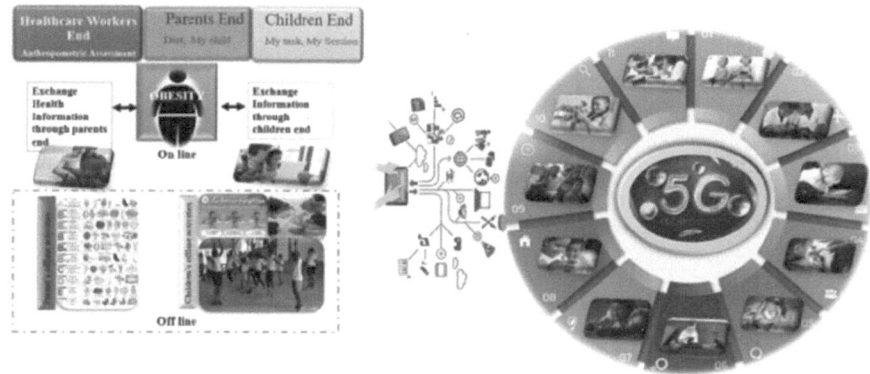

FIGURE 9.4 5G supported mobile games engaging children's.

develop a health application with three different modules. The first module can be for health care workers where they can collect and analyze the anthropometric data on a yearly basis. The second module can provide health information for caretakers who purchase and prepare foods and snacks for their children. The third module is the game module for children where they can learn about healthy food habits and play games physically to increase their PA as shown in Figure 9.4.

9.11 CONCLUSION AND RECOMMENDATIONS FOR FUTURE RESEARCH

Personal health behaviors are the major contributors to the health and wellbeing of the person. These behaviors can be cultivated early in the life of the individual and become sustainable if these behaviors are taught from childhood. Childhood obesity is easily preventable if early interventions are followed appropriately. Policymakers and health care workers are mainly looking for interventions that encourage positive health behavior change, particularly interventions using the skills of computing technology. Compared to the traditional methods, gamification has shown a new alternative model for health care. Due to the widespread use of mobile phones, laptops, and so forth, the potential to use gamification in the control and prevention of obesity is enormous. With the increase in 5G network coverage the potential to use gamification increases many times. The mobile applications can not only be used to deliver health-related messages and the physical activity components of any of the programs but can also be used to collect, compile, analyze and access the data easily at the click of the button.

The major setback in PICTs is the lack of availability of childhood obesity prevalence data which to some extend can be solved by using the appropriate mobile applications in a skilled way. The recommendation for future research involves the use of longitudinal studies by using large samples which can clearly show the effect of using gamification to enhance intrinsically motivated behavior. The mobile games used in different parts of the world need to be tailor-made to different regions as the availability and preparation of the food items are different in different places.

REFERENCES

1. Puska, P., and Nishida, C. "Obesity and overweight facts," *WORLD Heal. Organ. Glob. Strateg. DIET, Phys. Act. Heal.*, vol. 420, no. 13, pp. 6–18, 1980.
2. Cawley, J. "The economics of childhood obesity," *Heal. Aff*, vol. 29, no. 3, pp. 364–371, 2010.
3. Ogden, C. L., Carroll, M. D., Curtin, L. R., McDowell, M. A., Tabak, C. J., and Flegal, K. M. "Prevalence of overweight and obesity in the United States, 1999–2004," *J. Am. Med. Assoc.*, vol. 295, no. 13, pp. 1549–1555, 2006.
4. Florence, C., and Joski, P. "The impact of obesity on rising medical spending," *Health Aff.*, vol. Web Exclusive, no. 4, pp. 480–486, 2004.
5. WHO, "Global Action Plan for the Prevention and Control of NCDs 2013–2020," p. 103p, 2020.
6. Kelishadi, R. "A systematic review on strategies and challenges," *J Res Med Sci*, vol. 19, no. 10, pp. 993–1008, 2014.

7. Wolfswinkel, C., Furtmueller, J., and Wilderom, E. "Using grounded theory as a method for rigorously reviewing literature," *Eur. J. Inf. Syst.*, vol. 22, pp. 45–55, 2013.

8. Zhao, A., Ali, Z. S., and Arya, A. "Motivational impacts and sustainability analysis of a wearable-based gamified exercise and fitness system," in *2016 Annual Symposium on Computer-Human Interaction in Play Companion Extended Abstracts*, pp. 1–8, 2016. https://dl.acm.org/doi/10.1145/2968120.2987726

9. Webb, J., Eves, O. J., and Kerr, F. F. "Institutional repository a statistical summary of," *J. Phys. Act. Health*, vol. 8, no. 4, pp. 558–565, 2011, [Online].

10. World Health Organization, "Population-based Prevention Strategies for Childhood Obesity: a report of a WHO forum and technical meeting, Geneva 15–17 December 2009," 2010. [Online].

11. Krassas, G. E., Tzotzas, T., Tsametis, C., and Konstantinidis, T. "Prevalence and trends in overweight and obesity among children and adolescents in Thessaloniki, Greece," *J. Pediatr. Endocrinol. Metab.*, vol. 14, Suppl 5, pp. 1319–1326; discussion 1365. PMID: 11964029, 2001.

12. de Onis, M. "Development of a WHO growth reference for school-aged children and adolescents," *Bull. World Health Organ.*, vol. 85, no. 9, pp. 660–667, Sep. 2007.

13. Barlow, S. E., and Dietz, W. H. "Obesity evaluation and treatment: Expert committee recommendations," *Pediatrics*, vol. 102, no. 3, pp. e29–e29, Sep. 1998.

14. Stensel, S., Gorely, D., and Biddleg, T. "Youth Health Outcomes.," in A. L. Smith and S. Biddle (Eds.), *Youth Physical and Sedentary Behavior: Challenges and Solutions: Champaign, IL Human Kinetics*, p. 491, 2008.

15. P. R. C. for the P. of O. and NCDs., "Situational Analysis of Child BMI Monitoring in the Pacific Islands and Territories," no. December 2015.

16. Wilken, L. R., *et al.*, "Children's Healthy Living (CHL) Program for remote under-served minority populations in the Pacific region: rationale and design of a community randomized trial to prevent early childhood obesity," *BMC Public Health*, vol. 13, no. 1, p. 944, Dec. 2013.

17. Li, F., *et al.*, "Anthropometric measurement standardization in the US-affiliated pacific: Report from the Children's Healthy Living Program," *Am. J. Hum. Biol.*, vol. 28, no. 3, pp. 364–371, 2016.

18. Petersen, S., Moodie, M., Mavoa, H., Waqa, G., Goundar, R., and Swinburn, B. "Relationship between overweight and health-related quality of life in secondary school children in Fiji: Results from a cross-sectional population-based study," *Int. J. Obes.*, vol. 38, no. 4, pp. 539–546, 2014.

19. Ng, M. *et al.*, "Global, regional, and national prevalence of overweight and obesity in children and adults during 1980–2013: A systematic analysis for the Global Burden of Disease Study 2013," *Lancet*, vol. 384, no. 9945, pp. 766–781, Aug. 2014.

20. F. National Food and Nutrition Centre, "Fijian National Nutrition Survey 2016," 2016.

21. Davison, K. K. and Birch, L. L. "Childhood overweight: A contextual model and recommendations for future research," *Obes. Rev.*, vol. 2, no. 3, pp. 159–171, 2001.

22. Gauthier, K. I., and Krajicek, M. J. "Obesogenic environment: A concept analysis and pediatric perspective," *J. Spec. Pediatr. Nurs.*, vol. 18, no. 3, pp. 202–210, Jul. 2013.

23. Moreno. L. A., and Rodríguez, G. "Dietary risk factors for development of childhood obesity," *Curr. Opin. Clin. Nutr. Metab. Care*, vol. 10, no. 3, pp. 336–341, May 2007.

24. Bhuiyan, M. U., Zaman, S. and Ahmed, T. "Risk factors associated with overweight and obesity among urban school children and adolescents in Bangladesh: A case-control study," *BMC Pediatr.*, vol. 13, no. 1, 2013.

25. Patrick, H., and Nicklas, T. A. "A review of family and social determinants of children's eating patterns and diet quality," *J. Am. Coll. Nutr.*, vol. 24, no. 2, pp. 83–92, Apr. 2005.

26. Niehoff, V. "Childhood obesity: A call to action," *Bariatr. Nurs. Surg. Patient Care*, vol. 4, no. 1, pp. 17–23, Mar. 2009.

27. Daniels, S. R. "The consequences of childhood overweight and obesity," *Futur. Child.*, vol. 16, no. 1, pp. 47–67, 2006.

28. Franks, L. H., Hanson, P. W., Knowler, R. L., Sievers, W. C., and Bennett, M. L. "Childhood obesity, other cardiovascular risk factors, and premature death.," *N. Engl. J. Med.*, vol. 362, no. 19, pp. 1841; author reply 1841-2, May 2010.

29. Trasande, L., Liu, Y., Fryer, G., and Weitzman, M. "Effects of childhood obesity on hospital care and costs, 1999–2005," *Health Aff.*, vol. 28, no. Supplement 1, pp. w751–w760, Jan. 2009.

30. Schwimmer, J. B., Burwinkle, T. M., and Varni, M. W. J. "Health-Related Quality of Life of Severely Obese Children and Adolescents," 2003. https://jamanetwork.com/journals/jama/fullarticle/196343

31. Strauss, R. S. "Childhood Obesity and Self-Esteem," 2000. https://pubmed.ncbi.nlm.nih.gov/10617752/

32. Viner, R. M. and Cole, T. J. "Adult socioeconomic, educational, social, and psychological outcomes of childhood obesity: A national birth cohort study," *Br. Med. J.*, vol. 330, no. 7504, pp. 1354–1357, 2005.

33. Johnson, D. Deterding, S., Kuhn, K. A., Staneva, A. Stoyanov, S., and Hides, L. "Gamification for health and wellbeing: A systematic review of the literature," *Internet Interv.*, vol. 6, pp. 89–106, 2016.

34. Teixeira, P. J., Palmeira, A. L., and Vansteenkiste, M. "The role of self-determination theory and motivational interviewing in behavioral nutrition, physical activity, and health: an introduction to the IJBNPA special series," *Int. J. Behav. Nutr. Phys. Act.*, vol. 9, no. 1, p. 17, 2012.

35. Calvo, R. A., and Peters, D. *Positive Computing: Technology for Well-Being and Human Potential*. The MIT Press, ISBN: 9780262325684, 2014.

36. Fogg, B. J. *Persuasive Technology*. Elsevier, pp. 1–253, 2003.

37. Almonani, E., Husain, W., San, O. Y., Almomani, A., and Al-Betar, M. "Mobile game approach to prevent childhood obesity using persuasive technology," *2014 Int. Conf. Comput. Inf. Sci. ICCOINS 2014–A Conf. World Eng. Sci. Technol. Congr. ESTCON 2014–Proc.*, no. June, 2014.

38. Wright, J. K. "Pacific Islands," *Geogr. Rev.*, vol. 32, no. 3, p. 481, 2019.

39. Deterding, S., Dixon, D., Khaled, R., and Nacke, L. "From game design elements to gamefulness: Defining 'gamification,'" *Proc. 15th Int. Acad. MindTrek Conf. Envisioning Futur. Media Environ. MindTrek 2011*, pp. 9–15, 2011.

40. Sailer, M., Hense, J., Mandl, H., and Klevers, M. "Gamification as an innovative approach to foster motivation," *Interact. Des. Archit. J. - IxD&A*, no. 19, pp. 28–37, 2013.

41. Berger, V., and Schrader, U. "Fostering sustainable nutrition behavior through gamification," *Sustain.*, vol. 8, no. 1, pp. 1–15, 2016.

42. S. Editor Nilmini Wickramasinghe Epworth HealthCare Richmond, *Delivering Superior Health and Wellness Management with IoT and Analytics*. Cham: Springer International Publishing, 2020.

43. Deterding, S. "The Lens of Intrinsic Skill Atoms: A Method for Gameful Design," *Human–Computer Interact.*, vol. 30, no. 3–4, pp. 294–335, May 2015.

44. King, D., Greaves, F., Exeter, C., and Darzi, A. "'Gamification': Influencing health behaviours with games," *J. R. Soc. Med.*, vol. 106, no. 3, pp. 76–78, 2013.

45. Seaborn, K. and Fels, D. I. "Gamification in theory and action: A survey," *Int. J. Hum. Comput. Stud.*, vol. 74, pp. 14–31, Jul. 2015.

46. Oinas-Kukkonen, H., and Harjumaa, M. "Persuasive systems design: Key issues, process model, and system features," *Commun. Assoc. Inf. Syst.*, vol. 24, no. 1, pp. 485–500, 2009.

47. Lister, C., West, J. H., Cannon, B., Sax, T. and Brodegard, D. "Just a fad? Gamification in health and fitness apps," *JMIR Serious Games*, vol. 2, no. 2, p. e9, Aug. 2014.

48. Gurova, O., Merritt, T. R., Papachristos, E., and Vaajakari, J. "Sustainable solutions for wearable technologies: Mapping the product development life cycle," *Sustain.*, vol. 12, no. 20, pp. 1–26, 2020.

49. Zhao, Z., Ali Etemad, S., and Arya, A. "Gamification of Exercise and Fitness using Wearable Activity Trackers," in P. Chung, A. Soltoggio, C. W. Dawson, Q. Meng, and M. Pain (Eds.), *Advances in Intelligent Systems and Computing*, Springer, pp. 233–240, 2016, https://link.springer.com/book/10.1007/978-3-319-24560-7

50. Spil, T., Sunyaev, A., Thiebes, S., and Van Baalen, R. "The Adoption of Wearables for a Healthy Lifestyle: Can Gamification Help?" in *Proceedings of the 50th Hawaii International Conference on System Sciences (2017)*, pp. 3617–3626, 2017.

51. T. B. R. Company, "Smart Wearables Global Market Report 2020–30: Covid 19 Growth and Change," 2020. [Online].

52. Schulz, L., Ton Spil, A. A., and Snored de Vries, S. "Gamified wearables in obesity therapy for youth – Successful Fundamental app design guidelines," 2017.

53. Kayli's, A., Islas, T., Bergstrom, J., and Gore-Felton, C. "A review of efficacious technology-based weight-loss interventions: five key components.," *Telemed. J. E. Health.*, vol. 16, no. 9, pp. 931–938, 2010.

54. Baranowski, T., Buday, R., Thompson, D., Lyons, E. J., Lu, A. S., and Baranowski, J. "Developing games for health behavior change: Getting started," *Games Health J.*, vol. 2, no. 4, pp. 183–190, Aug. 2013.

55. Baranowski, T., Ryan, C., and Lu, A. S. "Nutrition education and dietary behavior change games: A scoping review," vol. 8, no. 3, 2019.

56. Baranowski, T., Buday, R., Thompson, D. I., and Baranowski, J. "Playing for real," *Am. J. Prev. Med.*, vol. 34, no. 1, pp. 74–82.e10, Jan. 2008.

57. Turning, M. C., *et al.*, "Evaluation of microcomputer nutritional teaching games in 1,876 children at school.," *Diabetes Metab.*, vol. 27, no. 4 Pt 1, pp. 459–64, Sep. 2001, [Online].

58. Hermans, R. C. J., van den Broek, N., Nevermore, C., Otten, R., Ruiter, E. L. M., and Johnson-Glenberg, M. C. "Feed the alien! The effects of a nutrition instruction game on children's nutritional knowledge and food intake," *Games Health J.*, vol. 7, no. 3, pp. 164–174, Jun. 2018.

59. Evans, C. E. L., Christian, M. S., Cleghorn, C. L., Greenwood, D. C., and Cade, J. E. "Systematic review and meta-analysis of school-based interventions to improve daily fruit and vegetable intake in children aged 5 to 12 y 1–3," pp. 889–901, 2012.

60. Vaziani, L-A., *et al.*, "Efficacy of school-based interventions aimed at decreasing sugar-sweetened beverage consumption among adolescents: A systematic review," *Public Health Nutr.*, vol. 20, no. 13, pp. 2416–2431, Sep. 2017.

61. Ezezika, O., Oh, J., Daegu, N., and Boyo, W. "Gamification of nutrition: A preliminary study on the impact of gamification on nutrition knowledge, attitude, and behaviour of adolescents in Nigeria," *Nutr. Health*, vol. 24, no. 3, pp. 137–144, Sep. 2018.

62. Holzmann, S. L., *et al.*, "Short-term effects of the serious game 'fit, food, fun' on nutritional knowledge: A pilot study among children and adolescents," *Nutrients*, vol. 11, no. 9, 2019.

63. Wang, J. J., Baranowski, T., Lau, P. W. C., Buday, R., and Gao, Y. "Story immersion may be effective in promoting diet and physical activity in Chinese children," *J. Nutr. Educ. Behave.*, vol. 49, no. 4, pp. 321–329.e1, Apr. 2017.

64. Del Río, N. G., González-González, C. S., Toledo-Delgado, P. A., Muñoz-Cruz, V., and García-Peñalvo, F. "Health promotion for childhood obesity: An approach based on self-tracking of data," *Sensors (Switzerland)*, vol. 20, no. 13, pp. 1–28, 2020.

65. Lee, J. E., and Gao, Z. "Effects of the iPad and mobile application-integrated physical education on children's physical activity and psychosocial beliefs," *Phys. Educ. Sport Pedagog.*, vol. 25, no. 6, pp. 567–584, 2020.

66. Ni Murch, C., *et al.*, "A co-designed mHealth programme to support healthy lifestyles in Māori and Pasifika peoples in New Zealand (OL@-OR@): a cluster-randomised controlled trial," *Lancet Digit. Heal.*, vol. 1, no. 6, pp. e298–e307, Oct. 2019, www.devex.com/news/using-apps-to-target-better-childhood-nutrition-in-the-pacific-93338

67. Cornish, L. "Using apps to target better childhood nutrition in the Pacific," *Inside Development*, 2018.

68. Galy, O., Yosef, K., and Caillaud, C. "Improving Pacific adolescents' physical activity toward international recommendations: Exploratory study of a digital education app coupled with activity trackers," *JMIR mHealth uHealth*, vol. 7, no. 12, p. e14854, Dec. 2019.

69. Veatupu, L., Puloka, V., Smith, M., McKerchar, C., and Signal, L. "Me'akai in Tonga: Exploring the nature and context of the food Tongan children eat in Ha'apai using wearable cameras," *Int. J. Environ. Res. Public Health*, vol. 16, no. 10, p. 1681, May 2019.

10 The Role of Photonics for the Realization of Future 6G Communication Systems

Kamal Kishor Choure, Manisha Prajapat,
Ankur Saharia, Nitesh Mudgal, Manish Tiwari,
Puspa Devi Pukhrambam, and Ghanshyam Singh

CONTENTS

10.1 INTRODUCTION

The domain of data communication has expanded immensely in the last decade with the introduction of new technologies in the hardware as well as the software part of the communication system. Worldwide mobile data traffic has been growing at an exponential rate for the past two decades [1, 2], and developments in the telecommunications industry will continue for many years. Since the evolution of communication technology, the demand for data flow has expanded substantially, and it is expected to surpass petabytes in the coming few years. Whereas the 5th generation (5G) communication system is still in its early stages of implementation, it has

DOI: 10.1201/9781003368311-10

a number of drawbacks, including high data traffic, latency, secured communication, power-efficient system, increased number of users, intelligent systems, and global coverage, against which researchers from all over the globe have already begun work on the 6th generation (6G) system, which will include a number of innovations and technologies that (5G) and its predecessor technologies lack [3, 4]. Researchers have documented the requirements and possible 6G architecture in [5, 6]. Scientific investigators from all over the world are introducing cutting-edge technologies like intelligent systems such as artificial intelligence (AI)/machine learning (ML), quantum computing for quantum information processing, quantum communication for secured communication of information, blockchain, photonic-Tera-Hertz communication, the Internet of Everything (IoE), quantum machine learning and others as key technologies in the realization of beyond 5G (B5G) and 6G communications [7–12]. Figure 10.1 summarizes the evolution of different communication generations and the associated technologies.

The generation of the cellular communication system started in the year 1980 with the introduction of 1st generation (1G) communication. With a gap of every 10 years, the 2nd generation (2G) and 3rd generation (3G) were introduced in 1990 and 2000, respectively. The 4th generation (4G) emerged in the year 2010 with extraordinary

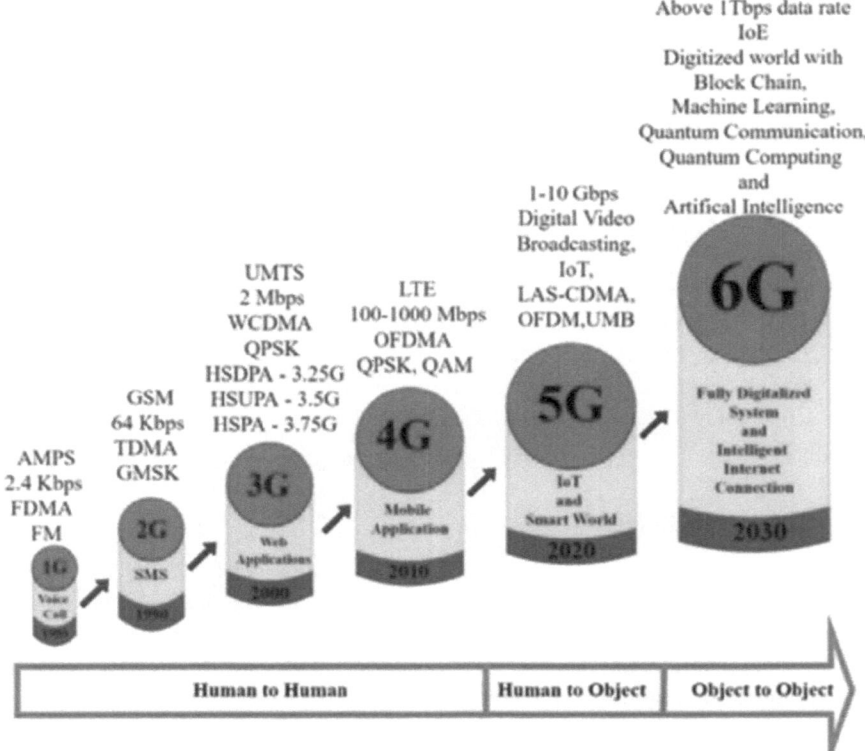

FIGURE 10.1 Evolution of different generations of communication systems.

facilities of internet data streaming, voice, picture, and video communication, online mobile gaming, internet banking, online shopping, the connection of smart gadgets, and the like. By 2020 some 5G communication came into the limelight showing some remarkable advancements. Still, there is a scope for improvement in terms of security, the implementation of intelligent connectivity, object to object connectivity, visible light communication, and so forth, which can be enhanced by 6G communication. The purpose of 6G is to fulfil the expectations of the communication system in ten years by 2030, which is much more than what 5G can provide [13]. In 6G "intelligent connectivity" comprises of intelligent interconnectivity among objects and network designs.

To meet the demands of future 6G communication, photonics provides the potential platform. Communication in 6G will be in terahertz (THz) and visible light communication (VLC), for which photonic devices can play a key role. Photonics technology has the distinct benefit of achieving a high modulation order by wave-mixing, high-speed amplitude, and encoding introduced by optical technologies. The high data rate of 6G communication can be achieved through THz communication by implementing photonics [14]. The integration of a large number of photonic components on a single chip provides the photonic integrated circuit. The key supporting technologies of 6G communication systems like AI, quantum computing, quantum communication, and THz communication are supported by photonic architecture for efficient performance.

10.1.1 KEY FEATURES AND PERFORMANCE INDICATORS

- In 6G the peak data rate is the main concern as by 2030 there will be lots of data-hungry applications introduced. It is expected to have 10 terabits per second data rate which is 10 times much more than the 5G communication data rate [2, 7, 14, 15].
- The second key performance parameter is global connectivity. It is likely to have cell-free communication with worldwide connectivity in 6G communication. In the 6G communication system there will be communication object to object with the associated IoE technologies, namely, a connection anywhere and at any time should be there for communication. As compared to a million devices per square kilometer for 5G, 6G is going to have 10^7 devices/Km^2 [2, 7, 14, 15].
- Efficient spectral utilization is one of the key aspects of 6G communication. It is predicted to have an intelligent network system in the future for educational organizations, hospitals, commercial offices, factories, and other smart gadgets with high extreme data rates which require a highly efficient spectral utilization. The 6G communication system is expected to provide 100 Bps [2, 7, 14, 15].
- ITU has proposed a mobility rate of >1000 Km/hr. for 6G communication. To avoid hindrances in communication while traveling in high speed trains and planes the mobility rate should be high for the 6G communication [2, 7, 14, 15].
- The possible 6G communication will be enabled with an advanced system such as a cell-free network, visible light communication, satellite integration, intelligent reflecting surfaces, and the like [2, 7, 14, 15].

- Until 2030 it is expected to have a large amount of data traffic because of the increase in wireless sensors, mobile, vehicular communication, and other AI-based gadgets for different applications to support this in 6G. The minimum area traffic capacity needed is $1000\,Mbps/m^2$ [2, 7, 14, 15].
- The expected latency rate for 6G communication would be <0.1 ms [2, 7, 14, 15].

10.2 ENABLING TECHNOLOGIES FOR 6G COMMUNICATION SYSTEMS

10.2.1 SPECTRUM TECHNIQUES

- **VLC:** The visual light communication range is 400 THz to 800 THz. This range of the spectrum is license-free and can be used without any limit, free of cost. In this range, there is no EM interference, and it can be implemented by using LEDs which are available at a low cost.
- **THz:** In the terahertz range, the bandwidth spectrum is high and the size of the antenna is reduced [16–20].

10.2.2 ANTENNA TECHNIQUES

- **Reconfigurable Intelligent Surfaces (RIS):** Reconfigurable intelligent surfaces are the artificial planar structures incorporated with an integrated circuit to manipulate the incoming electromagnetic signals. RIS antennas can be made small, can be controlled, and are also suitable for a programmable radio propagation environment.
- **Orthogonal Angular Momentum (OAM):** Orthogonal angular momentum antennas are used for obtaining a higher bit rate.
- **Lens Antenna:** In photonics, the lens antenna is extremely directive for high-frequency signal transmission [16–20].

10.2.3 PHYSICAL TECHNIQUES

- **Full Duplex:** This can be used for continuous transmission of a signal from transmitter to receiver and vice versa. It can be used in industry and for universal connectivity.
- **Out of Band Channel Estimation:** This provides more than one spectrum for flexible communication. It can be used in universal connectivity and in holographic telepresence.
- **Sensing and Localization:** These offer unique services and are managed using a context-based approach [16–20].

10.2.4 AIR INTERFACE TECHNIQUES

- **Massive Multiple Input Multiple Output (mMIMO) and Cell-free Massive Multiple Input Multiple Output (CF-mMIMO):** To increase performance, the number of elements in the antenna is increased in mMIMO. Whereas CF-mMIMO is used for removing inter-cell interference and enhancing the data rate at the cell edge.

- **Holographic Radio:** This provides more spatial multiplexing than mMIMO by creating a spatially continuous electromagnetic aperture.
- **NOMA:** Non-orthogonal multiple access methods are more efficient for higher multi-user capacity and for near-far effect [16–20].

10.2.5 NETWORK DESIGN TECHNIQUES

- **3D Network Architecture:** This is multi-connectivity and provides ideal services. It is also a cell-less architecture. It is deployed at a lower cost. This also provides advanced access backhaul integration and energy-efficient network operation.
- **Radio Access Network (RAN):** The advanced network slicing method improves the radio access network efficiency. The open radio access network is cost efficient and resource efficient.
- **Automation and Security:** Artificial intelligence and quantum computing methods help to make a system secure with high performance and lower expenditure [16–20].

10.2.6 INTELLIGENT NETWORKING TECHNIQUES

- **AI:** Networks that are used by artificial intelligence depend on machine learning and deep learning. Blockchain is also a decentralized, immutable, and transparent technology.
- **Quantum Computing and Communication:** To move towards a real-time environment, quantum computing is used. Quantum communication is more secure for communication networks [16–20].

10.3 PHOTONICS FOR 6G COMMUNICATION SYSTEMS

Photonic technology is electromagnetic interference-free and has high accuracy for high-speed optical signal processing. This topic has received a lot of attention lately, with new advancements pointing to photonic integration technology. Recent advancements in photonics technology could lead to a wide range of commercially sustainable 6G communication. Photonics devices are capable of handling and processing unparalleled volumes of data traffic with high energy efficiency, security, and low cost, resulting in new viable approaches [15]. The limits of electronic devices are overcome by photonic signal processing, which can accommodate multi-GHz sampling frequencies. As mentioned in [21–24] the all-optical phenomenon provides the extra cutting edge for optical and quantum computation. Figure 10.2 shows the wide range of photonic devices such as laser sources, optical amplifiers, optical switches, optical modulators, and optical passive devices that can be used to realize 6G communication [15, 24–26].

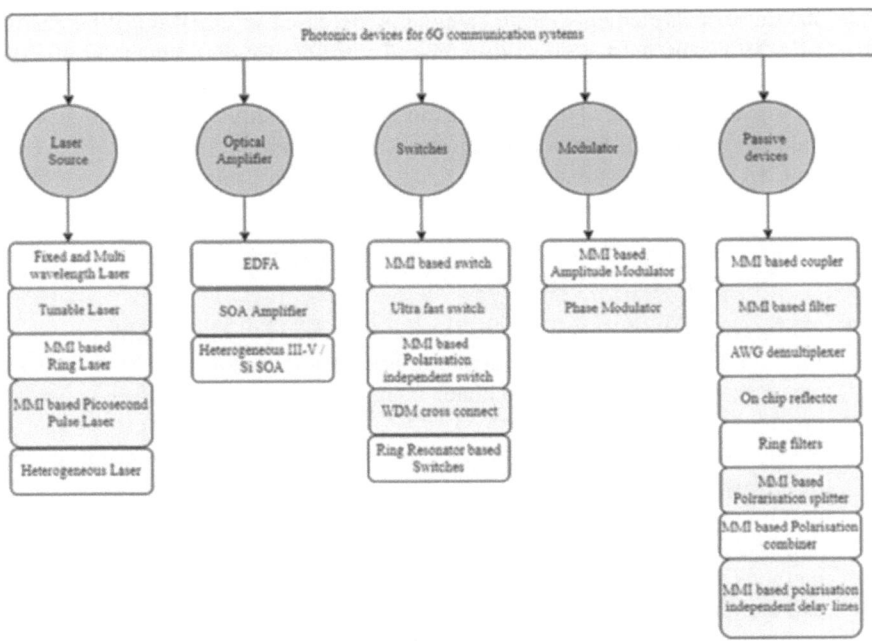

FIGURE 10.2 Photonic devices for 6G communication systems.

10.3.1 PHOTONICS COMPONENTS

The photonics components are the crucial partner in the implementation and real-ization of 6G communication. As proposed in [25] Light Fidelity (LiFi) and 3D imaging are door opening technologies for 6G. VLC, quantum communication, and LiFi-based communication are some of the key supporting technologies for 6G com-munication systems. Visual light communication (VLC), in which LED and laser sources are present, is best suited for 6G communication, because it requires high capacity, high speed, and high security. It also provides terrestrial, underwater, and space/air coverage for communication. The vital components of VLC, quantum com-munication and LiFi systems are optical components, for example, lasers, LEDs, optical modulators, optical amplifiers, optical detectors, optical filters, and optical multiplexers. Currently, indium phosphide (InP) optics and silicon photonics technolo-gies are employed to meet the requirement of VLC communication. The integrated photonic technology provides compact, high bandwidth, low power consumption platforms for the VLC system. A photonic circuit must be securely packaged and integrated with an external laser source. Silicon photonics technology combined with graphene materials will be able to perform different various optical operations such as switching, logic, routing, memory, and optical signal processing in 6G all-optical communication in the future. In designing amplifiers and lasers, heterogenous inte-gration of InP is used on a silicon wafer. Because just one PIC technology is used, heterogeneous integration of InP-Photonics on silicon platforms minimizes optical coupling losses and provides high-performance connections. Silicon photonics is driving an unprecedented technological shift in the optical network business, from discrete components to integrated chips. The silicon nitride (SiN) substrate can be utilized to make elements with minimum losses and wider fabrication constraints, and also improve thermal stability as mentioned in [24, 26–29].

10.3.2 PHOTONIC MODULATOR

Direct detection or coherent detection DWDM transceivers are used for different channel bit rates. Coherent detection is more efficient than direct detection because coherent detection provides a higher bit rate. For less complexity and low-cost intensity modulation-based channels, direct detection is used. Coherent detection is based on dual polarisation QPSK or dual polarisation 16-QAM [26–29].

Silicon-based Mach Zehnder modulators (MZM) are used for high bit rates. For modulation of the optical signal, Si PN junction-based phase shifters are used. In MZM for coupling of the optical signal, two Si grating couplers, which operate in C-band, are used [26–29].

10.3.3 OPTICAL AMPLIFIER

Erbium-doped fiber amplifiers are not compatible with photonic integrated circuits because in outdoor equipment, power consumption is critical. To reduce the size, provide low power consumption and low loss, SOA integrated with a silicon photonic circuit is used. By using an integrated amplifier, zero loss equipment can be designed.

Heterogeneous III-V/Si semiconductor optical amplifiers are used to overcome the loss at the transmitter and to amplify optical power at the receivers of the optical transceivers. At various wavelengths and input powers, the gain of the amplifier is obtained [26–29].

10.3.4 PASSIVE OPTICAL DEVICES, SWITCHES, AND MULTIPLEXERS

Passive optical devices are used for low cost, to simplify network operation, and to reduce equipment inventory. These filters are used in wavelength selective passive optical networks and broadcast-and select optical add-drop multiplexers.

The reconfigurable optical add-drop multiplexer (ROADM) provides flexibility in decreasing inventory cost, and network up-gradation, and enables software reconfiguration. ROADM can support 20 channels at the 100 Gbps bit rate and has less power requirement for wavelength selection.

Tunable photonics components such as filters, switches, and lasers can be implemented with the help of silicon photonics. Wavelength filters, switches, and modulators are designed by the thermo optic electro-optic effect in MZI and ring resonators.

Ring resonator based switching devices are designed for centralized access networks and are a prototype of the Mini-ROADM. The mini-ROADM device is polarization independent. To obtain polarization independence, a polarization diversity structure is used which consists of ring resonator-based switching elements.

TABLE 10.1
Recent Advancements in Photonics/Optical Domain for 6G

Author	Reported Work
Zhu et al. [30]	In VLC transmission, the 3D geometry-based stochastic model (GBSM) is to be preferred for indoor VLC channels which include characteristics of VLC such as space-time-frequency mobility caused by LED, high bandwidths, long paths.
Mostafa Zaman Chowdhury et al. [31]	Beyond 5G or 6G communication is based on IoT. Some essential issues are high capacity, more security, low power uses, and the like. RF networks alone are not able to reach our specification of 6G, so optical wireless communication (OWC) is used with RF networks that are compatible with 5G or 6G networks. In the future IoT tactile internet is become very useful for 6G communication.
Shintaro ARAI et al. [32]	The generation of mobile communication is enhanced almost every 10 years. The optical wireless communication (OWC) system is work on VLC or light fidelity (Li-Fi). This VLC range is suitable for 6G communication. Rolling-shutter method is used in cameras of mobiles and helps to obtain visible light beacon (VLB) identification.
Abhishek Gupta et al. [33]	In 6G communication VLC and the THz frequency range plays a vital role. In the VLC range, LEDs work for transmitting data. Even though LEDs are inexpensive and widely available, the influence of ambient light from other illumination sources, as well as sunlight, can be highly unpleasant and have numerous drawbacks. For 6G communication LED fulfils spectrum requirements and is an energy-efficient device.
A. Bigongiari et al. [34]	In 5G or 6G communication, a radio access network (RAN) is used in the range of millimeter waves. In advance antenna beamforming and spatial multiplexing technologies are being used. Remote laser source (RLS) is realized by two laser sources having orthogonal polarization. RLS is placed in the fronthaul link up to 3 kilometers, having 50 Gbps modulation format and placed up to 10 kilometers having 25 Gbps modulation format. This integration of RLS is energy efficient.
Nan Chi et al. [35]	In the next generation 5G/6G communication, the modulation scheme is enhanced, devices having new materials are developed, and the signal will be processed by artificial intelligence and machine learning. Almost all photonic devices are based on the VLC system.
Jiamin Gong et al. [36]	Jiamin Gong et al. proposed a Raman microstructure fiber amplifier for 6G. The proposed amplifier gives an average gain of 35.72 dB for 100 nm bandwidth.
E A Barabanova et. al.	This report presents high-capacity optical switches for 6G communication. The proposed switches have high throughput with low hardware costs.

A tunable laser is used for the obtained polarization-dependent loss at the input of the device [26–29].

10.4 CONCLUSION

To meet the requirement and realize the 6G communication systems, the photonics platforms can be potential platforms. Photonics has enormous advantages as compared to present electronics, which supports the implementation of 6G communication. The reduced size (nanoscale), low operating power, light weight, extremely large bandwidth, and compatibility for THz communication and VLC communication are some of the advantages of photonics.

Recent advancements also show that the photonics components can now be employed for AI, machine learning, quantum computing, and quantum communication which are the key enabling technologies of 6G communication. Still, there is improvement and advancement needed in the photonic transmitter and receiver section to provide the specific output for idle 6G communication.

REFERENCES

1. Zhao, et.al., "6G mobile communication network: vision, challenges and key technologies," *SCIENTIA SINICA Informationis*, vol. 49, no. 8, pp. 963–987, https://doi.org/10.1360/N112019-00033, 2019.
2. Liu, Q., Sarfraz, S., Wang, S. "An Overview of Key Technologies and Challenges of 6G". In: Chen, X., Yan, H., Yan, Q., Zhang, X. (eds) *Machine Learning for Cyber Security. ML4CS 2020. Lecture Notes in Computer Science*, vol 12487. Springer, Cham, 2020, https://link.springer.com/chapter/10.1007/978-3-030-62460-6_28
3. Chen, S., et.al, "Vision, requirements, and technology trend of 6G: how to tackle the challenges of system coverage, capacity, user data-rate and movement speed," IEEE Wireless Communications, vol. 27, no. 2, pp. 218–228, 2020.
4. Nawaz, et.al. "A review of vision and challenges of 6G technology," International Journal of Advanced Computer Science and Applications, vol. 11, no. 2, 2020, https://doi.org/10.1186/s13673-020-00258-2
5. David, K., and Berndt, H. "6G vision and requirements," IEEE Veh. Technol. Mag., vol. 13, no. 3, pp. 72–80, Sept. 2018.
6. Baiqing, Z., Xiaohong, Z., Jianli, W., Xiaotong, L., and Senlin, Z. "Photonics defined radio–A new paradigm for future mobile communication of B5G/6G," in Proc.6th Int. Conf. Photonics, Optics and Laser Technology, pp. 155–159, 2018.
7. Akhtar, M. W., Hassan, S. A., Ghaffar, R., et al. The shift to 6G communications: vision and requirements. Hum. Cent. Comput. Inf. Sci. vol. 10, no. 53, 2020.
8. Corre, Y., et.al, "Sub-THz spectrum as enabler for 6G wireless communications up to 1 Tbit/s," 2019, https://hal.science/hal-01993187/document
9. Nawaz, S., Sharma, S. K., Wyne, S., Patwary, M. N., and Asaduzzaman, M. "Quantum machine learning for 6G communication networks: State-of-the-art and vision for the future," IEEE Access, vol. 7, pp. 46 317–46 350, 2019.
10. Shafin, R., Liu, L., Chandrasekhar, V., Chen, H., Reed, J., and Zhang, J. C. "Artificial intelligence-enabled cellular networks: A critical path to beyond-5G and 6G," IEEE Wireless Communications, vol. 27, no. 2, pp. 212–217, 2020.

11. Xu, H., Klainea, P. V., Oniretia, O., Caob, B., Imrana, M., and Zhang, L. "Blockchain-enabled resource management and sharing for 6G communications," arXiv preprint arXiv:2003.13083, 2020.
12. Zhang, L., Liang, Y-C., and Niyato, D. "6G visions: Mobile ultra-broadband, super Internet-of-Things, and artificial intelligence," China Communications, vol. 16, no. 8, pp. 1–14 (P26-78), 2019.
13. Alsharif, M. H., Kelechi, A. H., Albreem, M. A., Chaudhry, S. A., Zia, M. S., Kim, S. "Sixth generation (6G) wireless networks: Vision, research activities, challenges and potential solutions. Symmetry, vol. 12, 676, 2020.
14. Yuan, Y., Zhao, Y., Zong, B., et al. "Potential key technologies for 6G mobile communications," Sci. China Inf. Sci., vol. 63, 183301, 2020.
15. Raddo, T. R., Rommel, S., Cimoli, B., et al. "Transition technologies towards 6G networks," J. Wireless Com. Network, vol. 100, 2021, https://doi.org/10.1186/s13638-021-01973-9
16. Jiang, W., and Schotten, H. The kick-off of 6G research worldwide: An overview. 10.36227/techrxiv.16552773.v1, 2021.
17. Giordani, M., Polese, M., Mezzavilla, M., Rangan, S., and Zorzi, M. "Toward 6G networks: Use cases and technologies," IEEE Communications Magazine, vol. 58, no. 3, pp. 55–61, March 2020.
18. Wu, Q., and Zhang, R. "Towards smart and reconfigurable environment: Intelligent reflecting surface aided wireless network," IEEE Communications Magazine, vol. 58, no. 1, pp. 106–112, 2019.
19. Faisal, A., Sarieddeen, H., Dahrouj, H., Al-Naffouri, T. Y., and Alouini, M-S. "Ultra-massive MIMO systems at terahertz bands: Prospects and challenges," arXiv preprint arXiv:1902.11090, 2019.
20. Hu, S., Rusek, F., and Edfors, O. "Beyond massive MIMO: The potential of data transmission with large intelligent surfaces," IEEE Transactions on Signal Processing, vol. 66, no. 10, pp. 2746–2758, 2018.
21. Minzioni, P., Lacava, C., Singh, G., Willner, A., Eggleton, B., et al. "Roadmap on all-optical processing", Journal of Optics, vol.21, no. 6, 2019.
22. Rachana, M., Swarnakar, S., Krishna, S. V., and Kumar, S. "Design and analysis of an optical three-input AND gate using a photonic crystal fiber." Applied Optics, vol. 61, no. 1, pp. 77–83, 2022.
23. Ankur. S., Maddila, R. K., Ali, J., Yupapin, P., and Singh, G. "An elementary optical logic circuit for quantum computing: A review." Optical and Quantum Electronics, vol. 51, no. 7, pp. 1–13, 2019.
24. Ankur. S., Mudgal, N., Choure, K. K., Maddila, R., Tiwari, M. Ghanshyam Singh, proposed all-optical read-only memory element employing Si3N4 based optical micro ring resonator, Optik, vol. 251, 168493, 2022.
25. Phichai. Y., Pornsuwancharoen, N., Suwanarat, S., et al. "High-density WGM probes generated by a ChG ring resonator for high-density 3D imaging and applications" MicrowOptTechnol Lett., vol. 60, no.11, pp. 2689–2693, 2018.
26. Chovan, J., and Uherek, F. Photonic integrated circuits for communication systems. Radio Engineering, vol. 27, pp. 357–363. 10.13164/re.2018.0357, 2018.
27. Iovanna, P., et al., "Optical components for transport network enabling the path to 6G," Journal of Lightwave Technology, vol. 40, no. 2, pp. 527–537, 15 Jan. 2022.
28. Sorianello, V., Testa, F., Velha, P., Doneda, S., and Romagnoli, M. "Experimental evaluation of residual added signal crosstalk in a silicon photonics integrated ROADM," in Proc. OFC, Paper Th2A.30, 2014

29. Menezo, S., et al. "Back-side-On-BOX heterogeneous laser integration for fully integrated photonic circuits on silicon," in Proc. 45th Eur. Conf. Opt. Communication, pp. 1–3, 2019.

30. Zhu, X. Wang, C-X., Huang, J., Chen, M., and Haas, H. "A novel 3D non-stationary channel model for 6G indoor visible light communication systems," IEEE Transactions on Wireless Communications, vol. 21, no. 10, pp. 8292–8307, Oct. 2022, doi: 10.1109/TWC.2022.3165569

31. Chowdhury, M. Z., Shahjalal, M., Hasan, M. K., and Jang, Y. M. "The role of optical wireless communication technologies in 5G/6G and IoT solutions: Prospects, directions, and challenges," Appl. Sci., vol. 9, 4367, 2019.

32. Shintaro, A. R. A. I., et al. "Optical wireless communication: A candidate 6G technology?" IEICE TRANS. Fundamentals, vol.E104–A, no.1 Jan. 2021.

33. Gupta, A., and Fernando, X. "Exploring Secure Visible Light Communication in Next-generation (6G) Internet-of-Things," 2021 International Wireless Communications and Mobile Computing (IWCMC), pp. 2090–2097, 2021.

34. Bigongiari, A., et al., "Integrated remote laser source for 6G advanced antenna systems," Journal of Lightwave Technology, vol. 40, no. 2, pp. 519–526, 15 Jan. 15, 2022.

35. Chi, N., Zhou, Y., Wei, Y., and Hu, F. "Visible light communication in 6G: advances, challenges, and prospects," IEEE Vehicular Technology Magazine, vol. 15, no. 4, pp. 93–102, Dec. 2020.

36. Gong, J., Liu, F., Wu, Y., Zhang, Y., Lei, S., and Zhu, Z. "Design of Raman Microstructure Fiber Amplifier for 6G," 2021 IEEE Wireless Communications and Networking Conference (WCNC), pp. 1–4, 2021.

11 MIMO Antennas for IoT and ISM Band Applications

*Inderpreet Kaur, Hari Kumar Singh,
Sanjeev Sharma, Navneet Singh, and
Yash Bhardwaj*

CONTENTS

11.1 INTRODUCTION

The Internet of Things will be authoritative, including a wide range of end systems, including smart homes, the engineering IoT, smart cities, smart agriculture, and smart networks. Aside from improved protocols of communication, antenna configuration will be a significant component related to smart devices that are node-end. Choosing the best antenna for work is an important planning task. Creating space for antennas is becoming a more difficult problem as IoT elements continue to become more

DOI: 10.1201/9781003368311-11

compact, integrating additional wireless technologies. As a result, antenna design for IoT modules must contend with the limits relating 'ever-shrinking' paths while retaining acceptable performance of antennas under important situations like fading, noise, and the need for efficiency. Improved techniques relating to scheduling, interference, multiplexing, and work related to radio resource allocation in tandem with antenna design helps to better understand capable antenna systems related to IoT. A key goal of this particular issue for new research is the growth of well-organized, scalable, cost-effective, antenna systems with reliability for the IoT. The effects of randomness in component locations in antenna arrays, MIMO antenna systems, MIMO system transference approaches, position tolerance design technique, and antenna designs related to ISM and RFID devices in an Internet of Things enabled environment, are all given special attention.

The Internet has changed the way we acquire data in the modern-day. More small gadgets with the ability to link to the Internet are being built as manufacturing prices fall, laying the framework for the IoT (Internet of Things). The major goal of the Internet of Things is to extend internet connectivity more than traditional devices like desktops and tablet to a wide range of other devices that use embedded technologies for communication and interact with one another over the Internet.

Increased channel capacity is possible using multi-input multiple-output (MIMO) systems, which do not require additional radio frequency spectrum and transmitter power. MIMO techniques offer a variety of benefits, including improved data rate, reduced multipath effects, and enhanced capacity, given the power and bandwidth limitations of the current generation of cellular systems. MIMO systems transmit and receive uncorrelated signals while improving channel capacity by generating parallel resolvable channels. The fundamental issues in MIMO antenna design are maintaining modest dimensions, good radiation efficiency, little envelope correlation, and great isolation between ports.

In a MIMO system, improper coupling between the radiating elements can dramatically increase signal correlation and reduce radiation efficiency. Exploiting pattern diversity to realize uncorrelated channels is one solution to this problem.

Antenna diversity is a technique for improving the signal quality and strength of an RF link by using several antennas. At the transmission point, the data is split into numerous data streams, which are then recombined on the receiving side by another MIMO radio with the same number of antennas. The receiver is programmed to account for the little time difference between the receipts of each signal, any additional noise or interference, and even lost signals.

Several types of research have been conducted in order to develop novel components and industrial technologies for future generations of wireless components and systems which are suitable for Internet of Things devices. Such devices show structures that meet IEEE research requirements for high data transmission, easy hardware components, consumption of low power, small sized, minimal interference, radiation patterns of omnidirectional type, phase response of linear type, amongst others. In 2002, the Federal Communication Commission designated industrial spectrum bands ranging from (3.1 to 10.6 GHz) for communication as well as data transfer. An antenna must have a wide bandwidth, decent radiation pattern, phase response of linear type, switchable capability as a front component of any wireless device, depending on the design characteristics. In UWB systems, the antenna response must cover the whole operating bandwidth, and transmissions outside the designated band should have no effect on the antenna. As a result, the antenna becomes the most important component in determining the performance of a communication system such as UWB. The narrow bandwidth properties related to microstrip patch antennas used to be a serious concern for researchers. The narrow bandwidth characteristics of 15–50% for general antennas in most wireless devices, such as dipoles and waveguide horns, were previously considered to be a severe constraint. There are various challenges for researchers to consider when it comes to antenna design. The majority of modern communication antennas have complex designs with uneven patch as well as dielectric substrates. Another important and difficult topic for antenna researchers to consider is antenna size reduction. The qualities of these sorts of antennas can also be affected by geometry related to mounting device upon which they are installed. It is now necessary to have a high bandwidth with a small antenna size and an easy design. In this study, authors present a structure for a compact 4-Port MIMO antenna related to applications for the IoT, with the key to obtaining a small size being careful design development while keeping acceptable electrical performance. By boosting signal quality, an MIMO system may improve system capacity, throughput, and QoS (quality of service), as well as reduce fading effect, lower tapping susceptibility, and improve system coverage. Microstrip antennas provide several advantages over other antenna types, including ease of fabrication, lower cost, multiband capability, small size, supports for both circular and linear polarizations, and the ability to be mounted on a hard surface. In microstrip MIMO antennas, surface waves play an important role in mutual coupling. In a MIMO system, there is a 'trade-off' between coupling and antenna size. Due to the restricted space, compact antennas having strong isolation are preferred for MIMO transmission. The effect of MC (mutual coupling) upon MIMO antennas has been studied in [1]. Many methods for decreasing mutual coupling for MIMO antennas were calculated in [2–4]. Researchers looked at a number of MC reduction procedures in order to attain the best MC. Some of the most common and widely utilized MC techniques are listed here. DGS (defected ground structures) may reduce MC by a level of 55 dB [5], resonator antennas having a dielectric may reduce MC by a level of 25 dB [6], CSRRs (corresponding split-ring resonators) may reduce MC by a level of 22 dB [7], lines of neutralization can reduce MC by a level of 23 dB [8–9], a slot element may reduce MC up to 22 dB [10], configurable antennas may decrease MC by a level of 47 dB [11], EBG (electromagnetic band gap) may reduce MC by a level of 53.7 dB [12], designed metamaterial may lower MC by a level of 42 dB [13], a decoupling network may decrease MC by a level of 32 dB [14]. DGS and EBG have been both effective methods for decreasing MC. For all meta surfaces, some meta surface innovations include the realization for different polarization-independent properties. UWB is a particularly desirable technology in a large no of applications, such as imaging systems, short-range radar, and wireless broadband applications [1–2], due to its high data rate, low power, and low cost. However, despite these benefits, UWB technology is plagued with transmission difficulties such as multipath fading. MIMO is viewed as a key to increasing channel capacity and lowering multipath fading in UWB systems without the requirement for more power [3–6]. More focus has been given to the development of a small 4-Port multi-input multiple-output antenna suitable for portable IoT devices. However, difficulties such as common coupling between nearby antenna parts develop when numerous antenna components are mounted on a receiving terminal in a compact space [7]. As a result, numerous novel techniques and procedures are recommended in literature to overcome this disadvantage while maintaining the overall size related to MIMO, using parasitic elements among antenna mounted substrates on both sides, that produce insertion losses of less than 20 dB in the band of operational frequency [8], and to reduce the mutual coupling impact, an arc-shaped defected ground structure is inserted in the base plane, and the value of common coupling may be suppressed for levels of 37.5 dB within the operating band among the antennas in [9]. [10] shows a different way of adding the neutralization line that improves the isolation between two similar antennas up to >25 db. A compact UC-EBG uniplanar electromagnetic band gap UWB MIMO antenna, with isolation superior to 18 dB throughout the whole impedance spectrum is also described in [11]. Multiple networks of narrowband wireless, such as 5G, having 3.6 GHz center frequency or Wi-Fi 6E having 6 GHz center frequency, may generate significant interference within the FCC-assigned radio spectrum of UWB (3.1–10.6 GHz). To alleviate this problem, band stop filter circuits may be incorporated into UWB devices, although this increases the cost and size of systems [12]. In [13–16], several UWB-MIMO antenna designs have been observed to exhibit band-notch behavior. In [13], a U-shaped slot is added on the surface of the antenna element to prevent current dispersion at 5.5 GHz. Two separate slits are loaded on each antenna element by the developers in [14] to give dual band rejection capabilities for Wi-MAX at 3.5 GHz and WLAN at 5.5 GHz. [15] produces a tri-band rejection concept by etching rotating C-shaped slots on the patches and rectangular shape slots on the base planes. Metamaterial structures (ELC) were used as a supplementary strategy for inducing notched resonance in the construction for UWB antennas [16]. SRRs and their related complements display LC resonator circuit behavior depending on their topology, and their permittivity and permeability are extracted with the use of Nicolson-Ross or transmission or reflection approaches [17]. The goal is to design planar antenna having a small footprint, low mutuality, and high multiband rejection.

The authors of this paper study a variety of EBG topologies on basic microstrip antennas in order to reduce mutual coupling (MC) among components for a 4-port MIMO antenna in IoT applications. This study begins using a 2.75 GHz design of microstrip antenna and progresses to a four-port MIMO antenna with no parallel slotted lines. The design and testing for a 4-Port MIMO antenna having a parallel slotted line between the pair of antennas are then planned, followed by a model of octagonal-shaped port construction [18–23].

All electromagnetic models and designs were approved using Ansys HFSS, a tool used in the simulation of three dimensional (3D) electromagnetics for high frequency constituents. Ansys HFSS uses a finite element method (FEM) to analyze HF (high frequency) devices such as antennas quickly and accurately. The suggested 4 PORT MIMO antenna has the following advantages and improvements [24–31]:

1. **Simplicity**: This framework is straightforward. It was designed and manufactured with low losses upon thin FR4-Epoxy substrate. It reduces the

complexity of systems, making it simple to integrate into a number of communication systems.

2. **Miniaturization:** By decreasing mutual coupling between the ports using a hybrid technique, the planned construction delivers higher performance in the industrial, scientific, and medical (ISM) frequency range in a compact size of $(40 \times 80 \times 1.6 \, mm^3)$.

3. **Virtual reflection coefficient:** The coefficient of reflection of the projected antenna being lesser than 1 dB over the whole frequency range. This coefficient shows that the impedance matching is better, and hence the power of radiation is sufficient.

4. **Less mutual coupling:** Over the full frequency or bandwidth range, the two sections achieve good isolation greater than 15 db. To accommodate a four-port MIMO antenna array into a tiny space, a multiple-parallel lines isolating device and a split octagonal ring resonator are used.

5. **ISM band application:** Electromagnetic interference is caused by the use of ISM equipment, which affects radio communications on the same frequency. As a result, this technique was restricted to a few frequency bands. Users have little influence over how ISM equipment is utilized since, in general, communication equipment operating in these bands should be able to withstand the interference created by ISM equipment.

6. **Novelty:** Combining an innovative technique, a multi-parallel line isolating element, CSRR and SRR were used in this paper for improving impedance matching, isolation, bandwidth, and for creating two innovative mechanisms using frequency band rejection, which is utilized for resolving electromagnetic interferences having two major applications with the involvement of the IoT and the ISM band range.

11.2 ANTENNA DESIGN

The geometry for a proposed 4-Port MIMO antenna having two frequency rejection characteristics is shown in Figure 11.1.

To provide a broad frequency response, design procedure begins with the fabrication of a four-port MIMO antenna having four symmetrical octagonal patches and a modified plane with partial ground. A four-line stub has been inserted at the plane with an upper ground over the entire bandwidth to improve bandwidth, impedance matching, isolation in-between the pair of elements of two antenna. To acquire our results within range of frequency of 2.25–3.0 GHz, CSRR has been imprinted upon the patch elements, and at the same time a SRR been loaded upon ground plane upon rear of every radiation element. The proposed structure was built on FR4-epoxy substrate having thickness equal to 1.6 mm, with ε_r (dielectric constant) equal to 4.4, tangent loss (δ) equal to 0.0023. The physical dimensions of the proposed 4-Port MIMO antenna, having the small size of 40×80 mm², are listed in Table 11.1.

Parameters	h	L	W	L1	W1	L2	W2	W3	R	R1	R2
Values (mm)	1.6	40.0	80.0	8.0	3.0	10.0	20.0	1.0	5.0	3.0	2.5

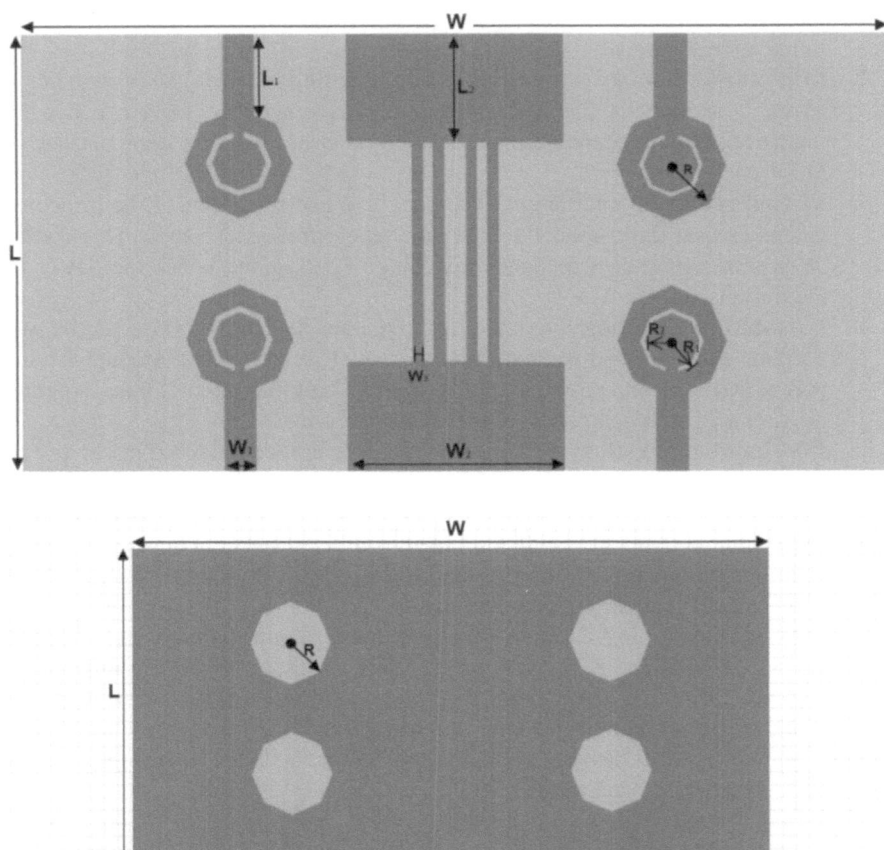

FIGURE 11.1   (a) Front part of the antenna, (b) Back part of the antenna.

11.3   EVOLUTION OF THE DESIGN OF COMPACT 4-PORT MIMO ANTENNAS

The design development of the intended Compact 4-Port MIMO antenna element is shown. The design process begins with the fabrication of an ISM band MIMO antenna using a modified partial ground plane and a traditional octagonal patch. The 10 dB impedance bandwidth of this setup ranges from 2.25–3.0 GHz, having low isolation throughout. Impedance matching, bandwidth, and isolation have all been improved with four-line stubs inserted in the upper half on the ground plane. Multi parallel lines serve like a resonator, generating transmission zeros between antenna pairs. The corresponding results reveal that the 10 dB bandwidth varies between 2.25–3.0 GHz. SRR is put on the base plane at the back side of the antenna, while CSRR has been mounted on the radiator patch to reduce signal interference in the ISM band [32–36].

11.4   DISCUSSION AND RESULTS

11.4.1   SCATTERING PARAMETERS FOR MIMO ANTENNAS

In the following subsection, the scattering parameters of the proposed Compact 4-Port MIMO antenna construction including the terms reflection coefficient, Z-parameters, and antenna to antenna isolation is discussed in depth.

11.4.1.1   Reflection Coefficient

The simulated and measured reflection coefficient plots for the suggested MIMO antennas are shown below. Some parameters of MIMO antennas are altered for isolation enhancement; hence MIMO antennas have a slightly different 10 dB bandwidth than the suggested single-element antenna. The antennas provide good impedance matching throughout a broad frequency range of 2.0–4.0 GHz, which corresponds to a fractional bandwidth of 15.9% with regard to the central operating frequency. Because all of the antenna elements have symmetrical form and location, the reflection coefficient curves are nearly identical. Due to measurement limitations, there is a small variance in the measured reflection coefficients among the antenna elements. The reflection coefficient (in dB) of the first port is shown in Figure 11.2(a) and the combined result of all the ports is given in Figure 11.2(b).

11.4.1.2   Z-Parameters

The Z parameter is used to determine an antenna's quality factor, which can provide information about the available bandwidth. $Z(ant) = R + jX$, where $R = R(rad) + R(Loss)$, hence the losses and efficiency can be predicted in some way. It could also be beneficial in identifying the equivalent circuit model of the antenna. The simulated and the measured Z-parameter plot of the proposed MIMO antenna is shown in Figure 11.3.

11.4.1.3   Antenna to Antenna Isolation

This antenna to antenna separation is a measure of how closely two antennas are coupled. Antenna isolation is typically evaluated for antennas within the same product, such as the separation between a smartphone's GPS and WiFi antenna. The isolation should be as large as possible when provided in this manner.

At the low band, isolation can be as low as −10 dB or less for antennas that share a similar ground plane, such as primary cellular antennas and the diversity on a smartphone. The efficiency of both antennas will suffer as a result of isolation. The simulated and the measured isolation plot of the proposed MIMO antenna is shown in Figure 11.4.

11.4.2   FAR-FIELD PARAMETERS FOR MIMO ANTENNAS

In the following subsection, the far-field parameters of the proposed compact 4-Port MIMO antenna construction include the terms 3-D Polar Plot, and gain that are discussed in depth.

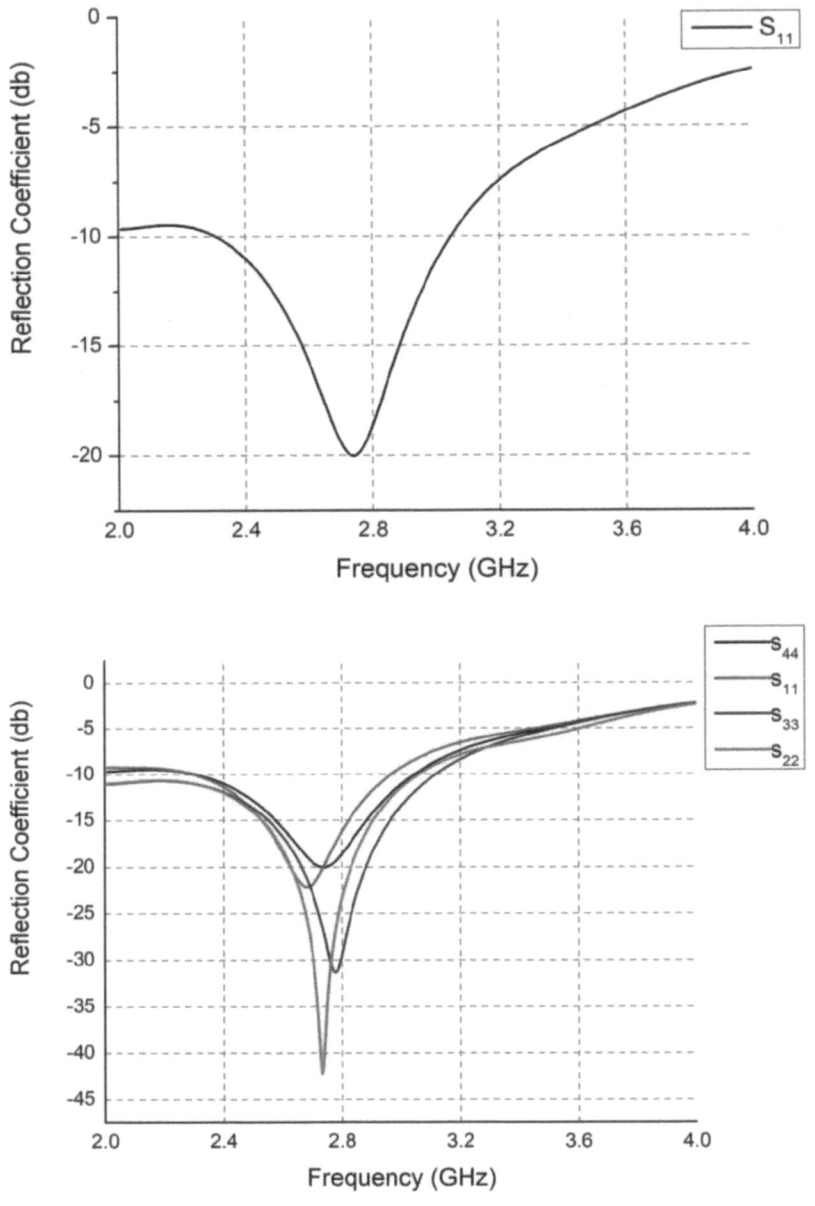

FIGURE 11.2   (a) Reflection coefficient of Port 1, (b) Reflection coefficient of all Ports.

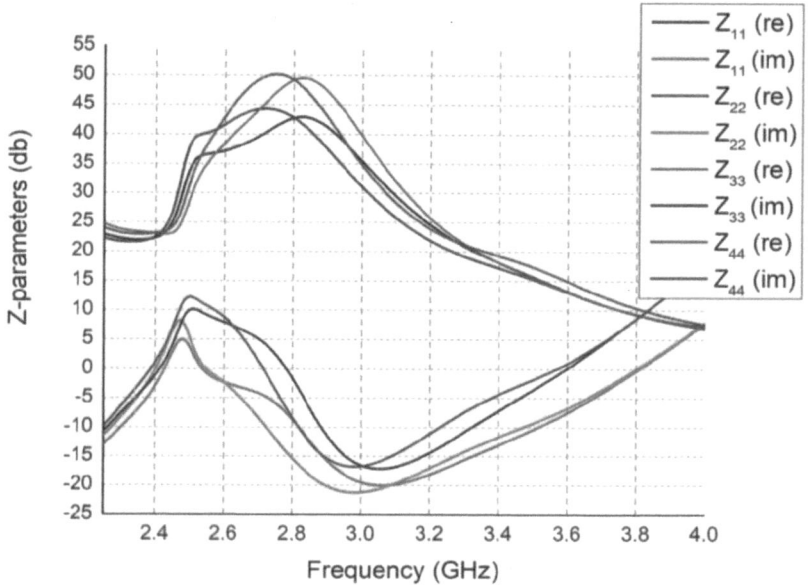

FIGURE 11.3 Z-Parameter of the proposed antenna.

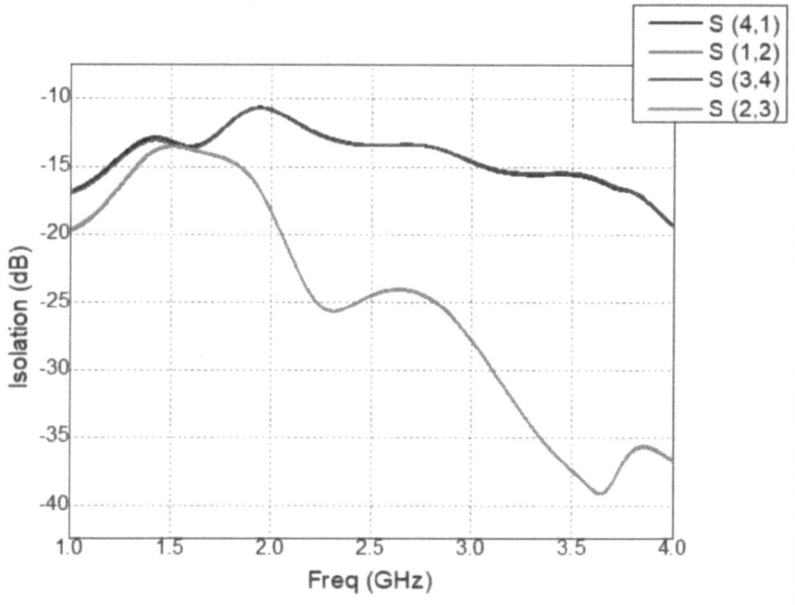

FIGURE 11.4 Isolation of the proposed antenna.

11.4.2.1   3D Polar Plot

The polar plot is a plot that depicts the transfer function of the system $G(j\omega)$ on a complex plane in polar coordinates. The polar plot representation depicts a plot of magnitude against phase angle in polar coordinates with variation in ω from 0 to ∞. The simulated and the measured 3-D polar plots of the proposed MIMO antenna are shown in Figure 11.5.

11.4.2.2   Gain

That portion of the radiation intensity in a given direction corresponding to a certain polarisation divided by different radiation intensity which can be obtained if the antenna's power was radiated in an isotropic manner. The total sum of the partial gains for any two orthogonal polarizations is the total gain of an antenna in a given direction. Losses due to impedance and polarisation mismatches are not included in the gain. If an antenna has no dissipative loss, its gain is equal to directivity in any direction. The direction of the peak radiation intensity is assumed if the direction is not provided.

The simulated and the measured gain plot of the proposed MIMO antenna is shown in Figure 11.6.

11.4.3   PERFORMANCE PROVIDING PARAMETERS OF MIMO ANTENNA

In the following subsection, the performance of the proposed compact 4-Port MIMO antenna construction including the terms DG, ECC, TARC, and efficiency is discussed in depth.

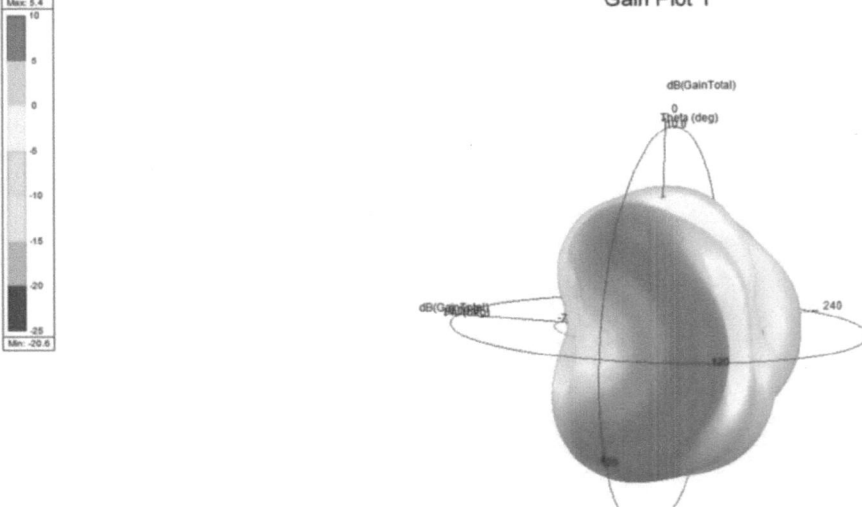

FIGURE 11.5   3-Dimensional polar plot of the proposed antenna design.

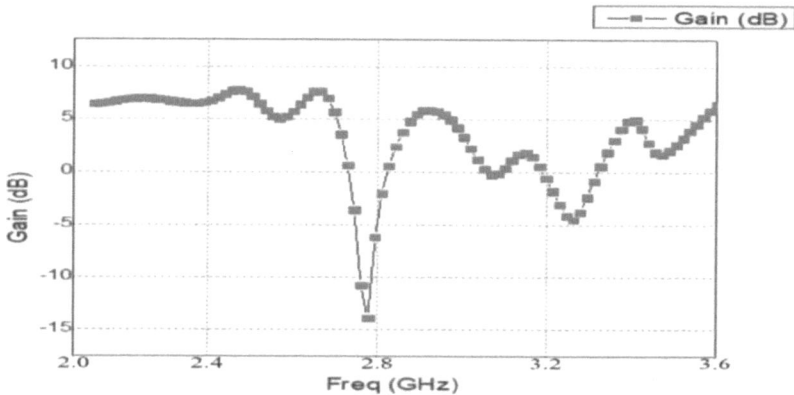

FIGURE 11.6   Gain plot of the proposed antenna.

11.4.3.1   Envelope Correlation Coefficient and Diversity Gain

The ECC between the ith and j^{th} radiation elements of an N port MIMO antenna system using far-field patterns is given by Equation (11.1).

$$
\mathrm{ECC}(i,j) = \left(\int\limits_0^{2\pi}\int\limits_0^{\pi} \left(\mathrm{XPR}\, E_{\theta i} E_{\theta j}^* P_\theta + E_{\varphi i} E_{\varphi j}^* P_\varphi \right) d\Omega \right) /
$$

$$
\left[\left(\int\limits_0^{2\pi}\int\limits_0^{\pi} \left(\mathrm{XPR}\, E_{\theta i} E_{\theta i}^* P_\theta + E_{\varphi i} E_{\varphi i}^* P_\varphi \right) d\Omega \right) \times \int\limits_0^{2\pi}\int\limits_0^{\pi} \left(\mathrm{XPR}\, E_{\theta j} E_{\theta j}^* P_\theta + E_{\varphi j} E_{\mathcal{A}j}^* P_{\mathcal{E}} \right) d\Omega \right]
$$

(Eq. 11.1)

where XPR represents the cross-polarization power ratio of the propagation surroundings. In the above formula, $E_\theta(\Omega)\ E_\theta^*(\Omega)$ and $E_\varphi(\Omega)\ E_\varphi^*(\Omega)$ are the power patterns of θ and φ polarizations, correspondingly. $P_\theta(\Omega)$ and $P_\varphi(\Omega)$ indicate the angular density functions of the θ and φ polarizations, correspondingly. $E_{\theta i}(\Omega)$ and $E_{\theta j}(\Omega)$ are the electric field patterns of the ith and j^{th} antenna elements in the θ polarization, in that order. $E_{\varphi i}(\Omega)$ and $E_{\varphi j}(\Omega)$ are the electric field patterns of the ith and j^{th} antenna elements in the φ polarization, individually. For uniform multipath environ-

ment, XPR = 1 and $P_\theta(\Omega) = P_A(\Omega) = \dfrac{1}{4\pi}$.

The following expression specifies the DG of the planned MIMO antenna [18]: $DG = 10\sqrt{1 - |\rho|^2}$

where ρ is the coefficient of complex cross-correlation, and $|\rho|^2 \approx$ ECC. Figures 11.7 and 11.8 show the ECC and DG graphs that were simulated and measured. The radiation patterns are used to generate the simulated ECC and DG results, while the S-parameters are used to generate the measured results.

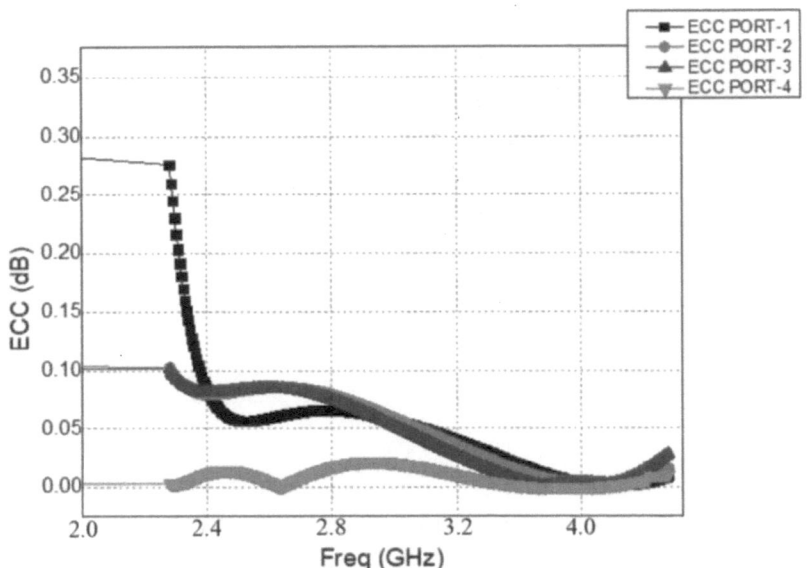

FIGURE 11.7   ECC of all ports of the proposed antenna.

As we can see from Figure 11.7, the ECC is less than 0.03 for the whole ISM band, except in the frequency band (3–4.4 GHz), where the ECC is greater than 1 db. As indicated in Figure 11.8, the DG is larger than 9.75 dB.

11.4.3.2 Efficiency

The high radiation efficiency of over 83% backs up the compact 4-Port MIMO antenna's almost constant performance.

11.4.3.3 Total Active Reflection Coefficient

For a four-port MIMO system, i = 1, 2, 3, 4, j = 2, 3, 4, 1 in that order and N = 4. The following equation considers the TARC using the S-parameters:

$$TARC = \sqrt{\frac{\left|S_{ii} + S_{ij}e^{j\theta}\right|^2 + \left|S_{jj} + S_{ji}e^{j\theta}\right|^2}{2}}$$

where the Gaussian random input feed phase is θ, and it varies from 0 to π. As seen in Figure 11.9, this parameter is less than -10 dB over the whole frequency range. The slight disparity between the simulated and observed findings could be related to the effect of soldering the SMA connectors, as well as the tolerance levels for the antenna construction process period.

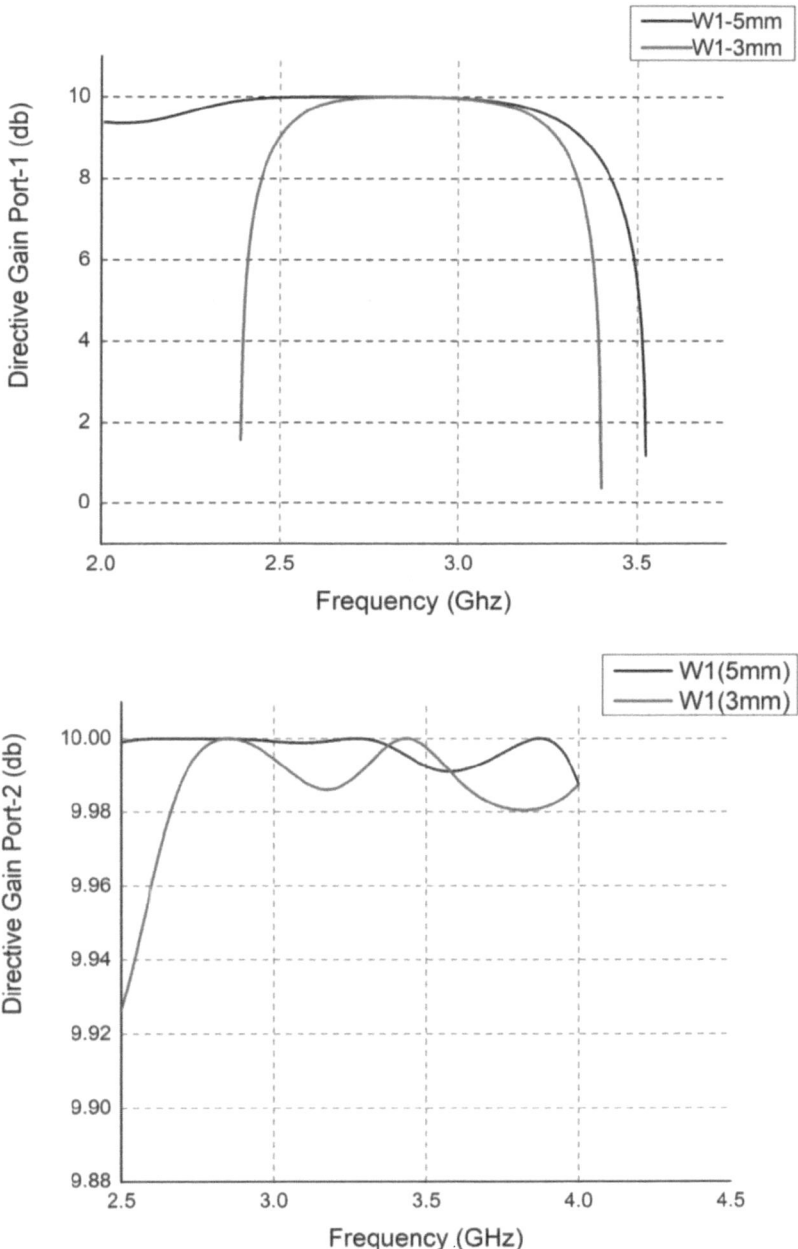

FIGURE 11.8   (a–d) DG of all ports of antenna.

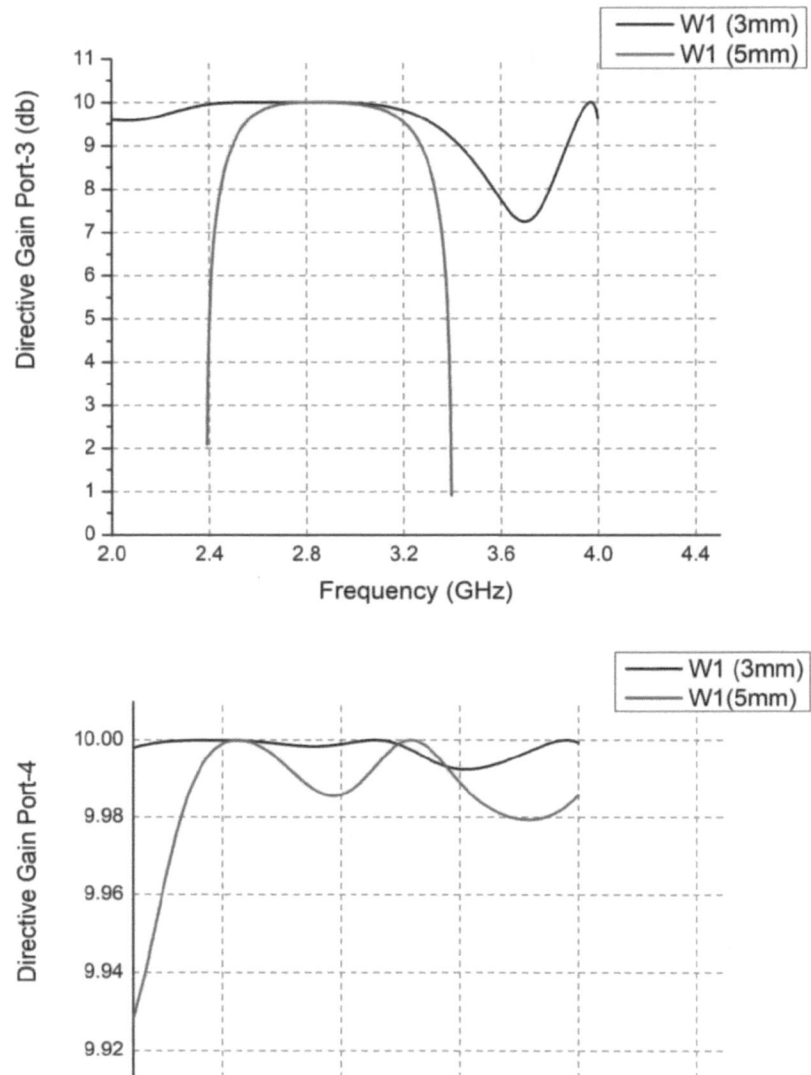

FIGURE 11.8 (continued)

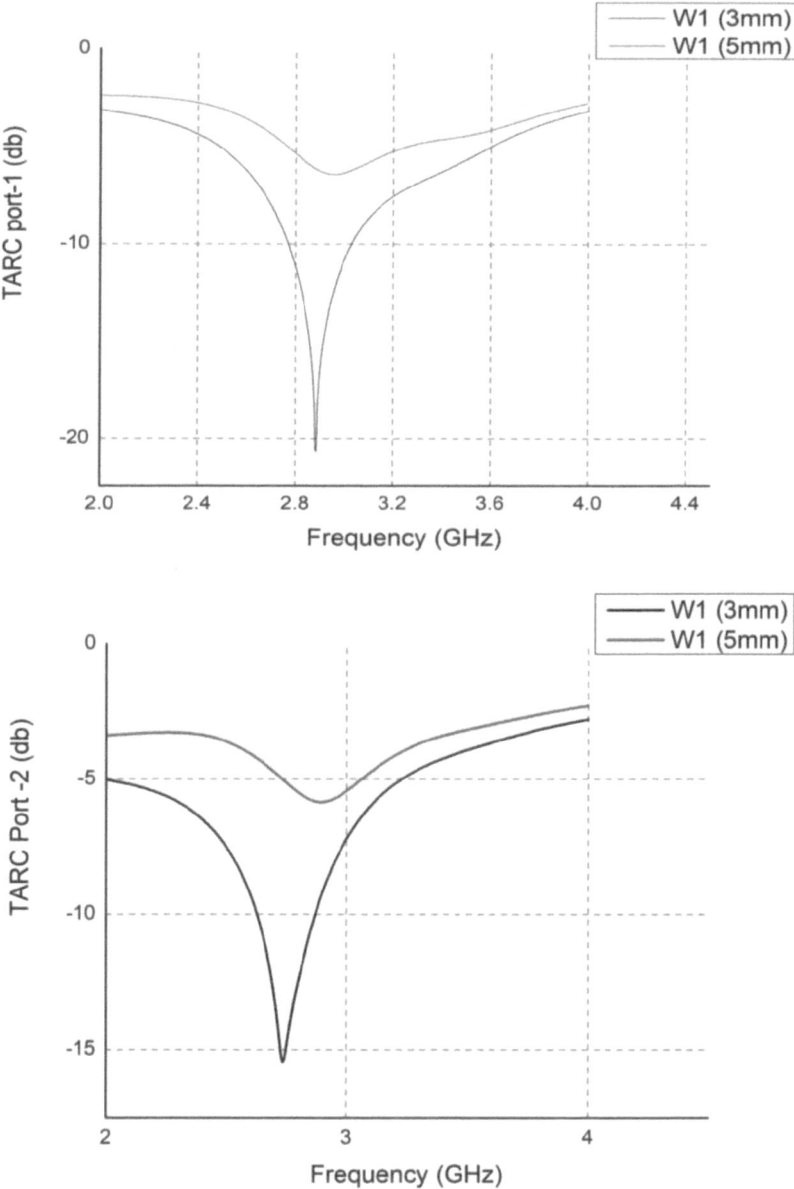

FIGURE 11.9   (a–d) TARC of all ports of the proposed antenna.

11.4.3.4   Voltage Standing Wave Ratio (VSWR)

The voltage standing wave ratio, or VSWR, is the ratio of a lossless line's maximum to minimum voltage. In actuality, any feeder or transmission line will experience a loss. To calculate the VSWR, forward and reverse power are detected at that

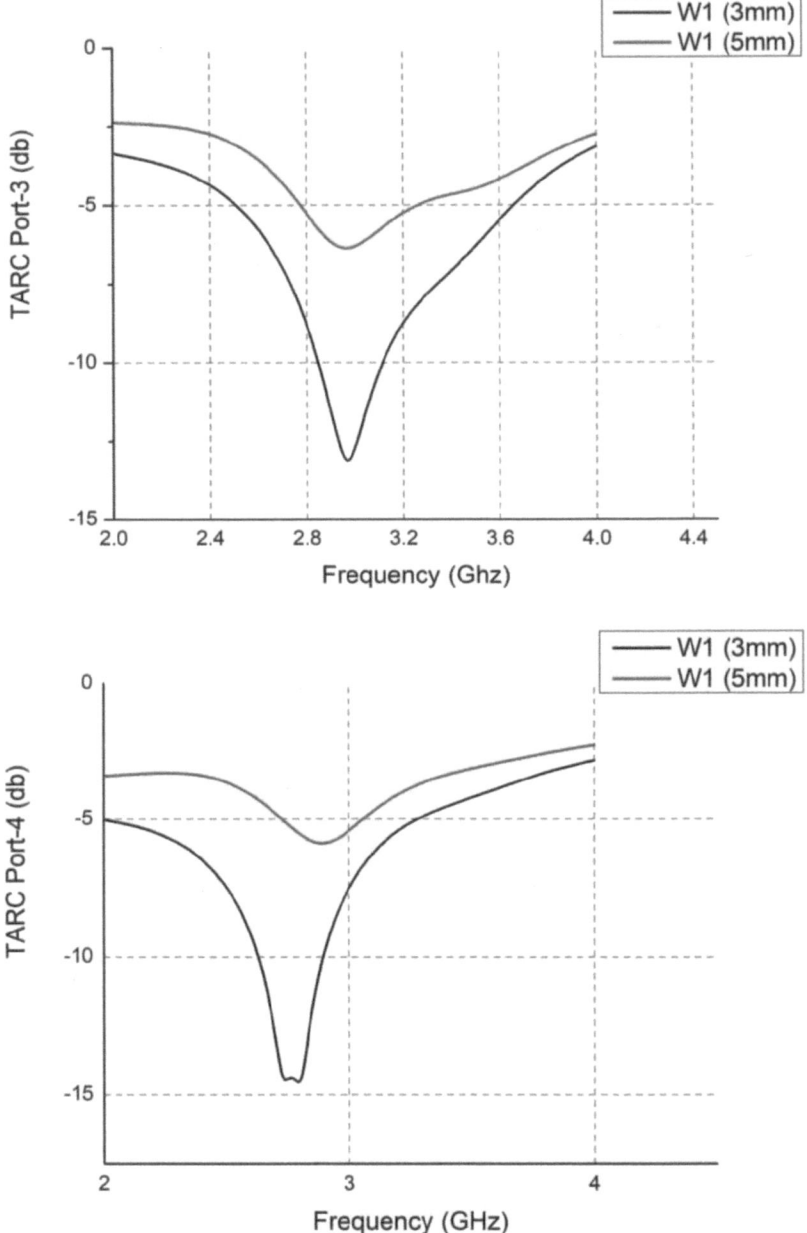

FIGURE 11.9   (continued)

location on the system and transformed into a VSWR figure. The voltage maxima and minima do not need to be determined along the length of the line because the VSWR is measured at a specific place. Figure 11.10 depicts the VSWR of all of the antenna's ports.

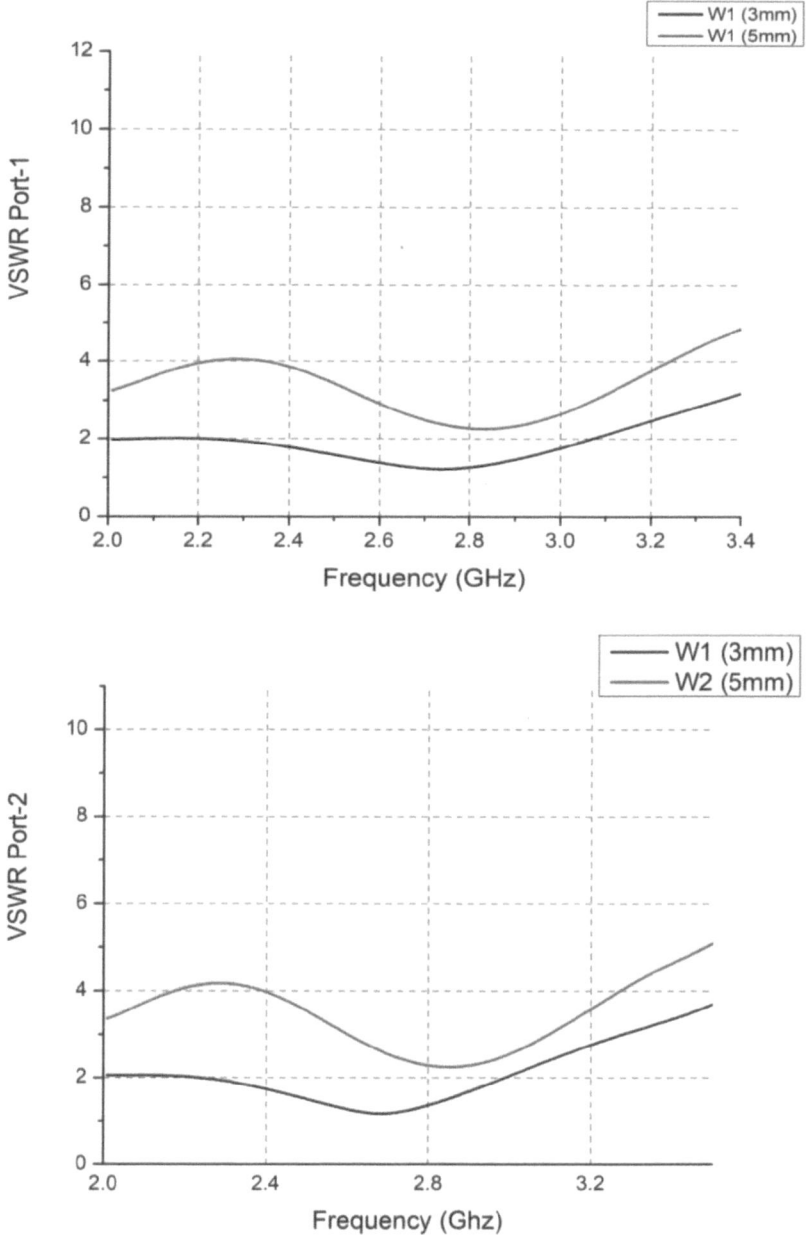

FIGURE 11.10   (a–d) VSWR of all ports of the proposed antenna.

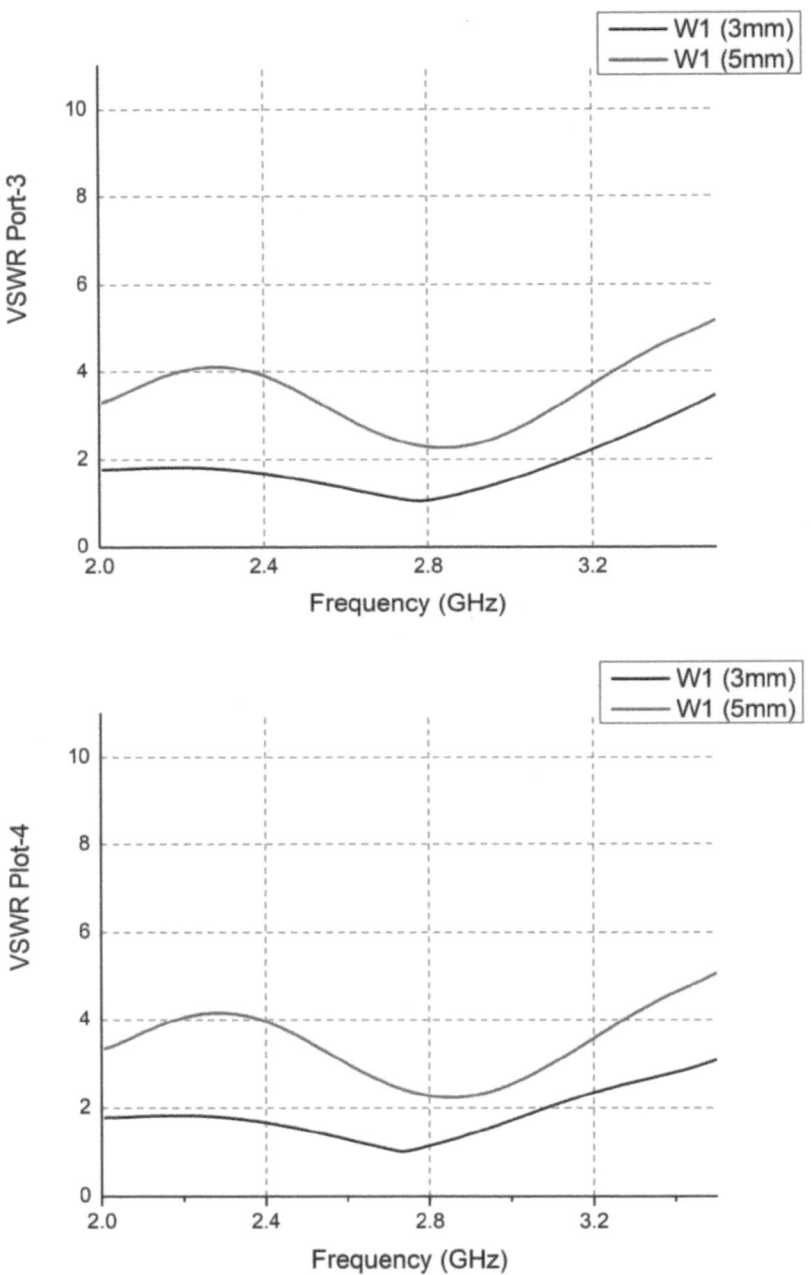

FIGURE 11.10 (continued)

TABLE 11.1
Simulation parameters

Ref. No.	Year	Number of Ports	Size (mm^3)	Isolation (dB)	ECC	Bandwidth (GHz)	Efficiency (%)	DG (dB)
[19]	2018	2	30 × 41	<-20	<0.1	2.2 GHz to 5 GHz	80	-
[20]	2018	3	58 × 45	<-15	<0.6	3.1 Ghz to 7 GHz	80	-
[21]	2021	2	50 × 50	<-21	<0.04	2.36 GHz to 12 GHz	-	9.99
[22]	2020	2	32 × 46	<-20	<0.5	3 GHz to 11 Ghz	-	-
[23]	2018	1	46 × 46	<-17	<0.02	-	75	-
[24]	2015	2	40 × 40	<-15	-	2.3 GHz to 8.8 GHz	-	-
[25]	2015	1	38.5 × 38.5	<-15	<0.1	2.5 GHz to 12 GHz	>75	99
[26]	2014	0	40 × 40	-	<0.005	2.2 GHz to 13.3 GHz	-	8-9.5
[27]	2021	2	48 × 48	<-18	<0.04	2.5 Hz to 5 GHz	-	-
[28]	2014	1	50 × 82	<-15	<0.02	3 GHz to 9 GHz	60	-
[29]	2017	1	40 × 30	<-15		2.2 GHz to 4.25 GHz	58	9.94
P.S	2022	4	×					

Note: P.S = proposed structure; DG = Directive Gain; ECC = Envelope correlation coefficient'.

11.5 PERFORMANCE COMPARISON

In terms of size, isolation between antenna elements, ECC, operating bands, efficiency, and DG, Table 11.1 compares the planned compact four-port MIMO antenna array to different existing MIMO systems. The proposed 4-port MIMO antenna has a wide impedance bandwidth, modest dimensions, and excellent ECC and DG values, as indicated in the table.

11.6 CONCLUSION

Antennas with pattern diversity for multiple input multiple output (MIMO) are a critical technology for modern mobile communication systems that enable excellent spectrum efficiency. The size of the device, which restricts the number of radiating parts, is a major limiting issue in this technology. This is owing to the fact that great plane isolation is maintained. This method ensures strong isolation between the ports and can result in directive patterns from each MIMO antenna element. As a result, the final design is ideal for pattern diversity. The technique is applied to an IFA antenna, and 4 and 6 element MIMO antennas are simulated and built to prove the validity of the suggested technique. The simulation and measurement agree well, which supports the validity of the suggested technique. This technology could be a suitable fit for designing huge MIMO antennas for IoT and 5G systems that demand a large number of antennas in a small space.

REFERENCES

1. Chen, X., Zhang, S., and Li, Q. "A review of mutual coupling in MIMO systems," IEEE Access, Vol. 6, 24706–24719, 2018.

2. Malathi, A. C. J., and Thiripurasundari, D. "Review on isolation techniques in MIMO antenna systems," Indian Journal of Science and Technology, Vol. 9, No. 35, 2016. [Online].

3. Chouhan, S., Panda, D. K., Gupta, M., and Singhal, S. "Multiport MIMO antennas with mutual coupling reduction techniques for modern wireless transceiver operations: A review," International Journal of RF and Microwave Computer-Aided Engineering, Vol. 28, No. 2, e21189, 2018.

4. Shoaib, N., Shoaib, S., Khattak, R. Y., Shoaib, I., Chen, X., and Perwaiz, A. "MIMO antennas for smart 5g devices," IEEE Access, Vol. 6, 77014–77021, 2018.

5. Wei, K., Li, J., Wang, L., Xing, Z., and Xu, R. "S-shaped periodic defected ground structures to reduce microstrip antenna array mutual coupling," Electronics Letters, Vol. 52, No. 15, 1288–1290, 2016.

6. Das, G., Sharma, A., and Gangwar, R. K. "Dielectric resonator-based two-element MIMO antenna system with dual-band characteristics," IET Microwaves, Antennas Propagation, Vol. 12, No. 5, 734–741, 2018.

7. Ramachandran, A., Valiyaveettil Pushpakaran, S., Pezholil, M., and Kesavath, V. "A four-port MIMO antenna using concentric square-ring patches loaded with CSRR for high isolation," IEEE Antennas and Wireless Propagation Letters, Vol. 15, 1196–1199, 2016.

8. Wang, S., and Du, Z. "Decoupled dual-antenna system using crossed neutralization lines for LTE/WWAN smartphone applications," IEEE Antennas and Wireless Propagation Letters, Vol. 14, 523–526, 2015.

9. Tiwari, R. N., Singh, P., Kanaujia, B. K., and Srivastava, K. "Neutralization technique based two and four-port high isolation MIMO antennas for UWB communication," AEU-International Journal of Electronics and Communications, Vol. 110, 152828, 2019.

10. Srivastava, G., and Mohan, A. "Compact MIMO slot antenna for UWB applications," IEEE Antennas and Wireless Propagation Letters, Vol. 15, 1057–1060, 2016.

11. Lim, J., Jin, Z., Song, C., and Yun, T. "Simultaneous frequency and isolation reconfigurable MIMO PIFA using pin diodes," IEEE Transactions on Antennas and Propagation, Vol. 60, No. 12, 5939–5946, Dec. 2012.

12. Lee, J., Kim, S., and Jang, J. "Reduction of mutual coupling in planar multiple antennae by using 1-D EBG and SRR structures," IEEE Transactions on Antennas and Propagation, Vol. 63, No. 9, 4194–4198, Sep. 2015.

13. Zhai, G., Chen, Z. N., and Qing, X. "Enhanced isolation of a closely spaced four-element MIMO antenna system using metamaterial mushroom," IEEE Transactions on Antennas and Propagation, Vol. 63, No. 8, 3362–3370, Aug. 2015.

14. Zhao, L., and Wu, K. "A dual-band coupled-resonator decoupling network for two coupled antennas," IEEE Transactions on Antennas and Propagation, Vol. 63, No. 7, 2843–2850, Jul. 2015.

15. Yuan, Y., Zhang, K., Ding, X., Ratni, B., Buroker, S. N., and Wu, Q. "Complementary transmissive ultra-thin meta-deflectors for broadband polarization-independent refractions in the microwave region," Photon. Res., Vol. 7, No. 1, 80–88, Jan. 2019.

16. Zhang, K., Yuan, Y., Ding, X., Ratni, B., Buroker, S. N., and Wu, Q. "High-efficiency meta lenses with switchable functionalities in the microwave region," ACS Applied Materials and Interfaces, Vol. 11, No. 31, 28423–28430, 2019.

17. Kim, K. H., and Schutt-Aine, J. E. "Analysis and modeling of hybrid planar-type electromagnetic bandgap structures and feasibility study on power distribution network applications," IEEE Transactions on Microwave Theory and Techniques, Vol. 56, No. 1, 178–186, Jan. 2008.

18. Su, S., Lee, C., and Chang, F. "Printed MIMO-antenna system using the neutralization-line technique for wireless USB-dongle applications," IEEE Transactions on Antennas and Propagation, Vol. 60, No. 2, 456–463, Feb. 2012.

19. Gorai, A., Dasgupta, A., and Ghatak, R. "A compact quasi-self-complementary dual band-notched UWB MIMO antenna with enhanced isolation using Hilbert fractal slot," AEU — Int. J. Electron. Commun., Vol. 94, June, 36–41, 2018.

20. Jaglan, N., Gupta, S. D., Kanaujia, B. K., Srivastava, S., and Thakur, E. "Triple band-notched DGCEBG structure-based UWB MIMO/diversity antenna," Progress in Electromagnetics Research C, Vol. 80, 21–37, 2018.

21. Zhou, J. Y., Wang, Y. F., Xu, J. M., and Du, C. Z. "A CPW-fed UWB-MIMO antenna with high isolation and dual band-notched characteristic," Progress in Electromagnetics Research M, Vol. 102, January, 27–37, 2021.

22. Zhang, J., Wang, L., and Zhang, W. "A novel dual band-notched CPW-fed UWB MIMO antenna with mutual coupling reduction characteristics," Progress in Electromagnetics Research Letters, Vol. 90, December, 21–28, 2020.

23. Debnath, P., Karmakar, A., Saha, A. and Huda, S. "UMB MIMO Slot antenna with Minkowski fractal shaped isolators for isolation enhancement," progress In Electromagnetics Research M, Vol. 75, September, 69–78, 2018.

24. Zhu, J., Feng, B., Peng, B., Li, S., and Deng, L. "Compact CPW UWB diversity slot antenna with dual band-notched characteristics," Microw. Opt. Technol. Lett., Vol. 55, No. 11, 2562–2568, 2015.

25. Kang, L., Li, H., Wang, X., and Shi, X. "Compact offset microstrip-fed MIMO antenna for band-notched UWB applications," IEEE Antennas Wirel. Propag. Lett., Vol. 14, 1754–1757, 2015.

26. Mao, C. X., and Chu, Q. X. "Compact radiator UWB-MIMO antenna with dual polarization," IEEE Trans. Antennas Propag., Vol. 62, No. 9, 4474–4480, 2014.

27. Mohan Reddy, S. S., Sanjay, B., Aruna Kumari, K., Madhav, B. T. P., and Prudhvi Nadh, B. "MIMO dual-sensing antenna with notch characteristics," J. Phys. Conf. Ser., Vol. 1804, No. 1, 012194, 2021.

28. Gao, P., He, S., Wei, X., Xu, Z., Wang, N., and Zheng, Y. "Compact printed uwb diversity slot antenna with 5.5-GHz band-notched characteristics," IEEE Antennas Wirel. Propag. Lett., Vol. 13, 376–379, 2014.

29. Toktas, A. "G-shaped band-notched ultra-wideband MIMO antenna system for mobile terminals," IET Microwaves, Antennas Propag., Vol. 11, No. 5, 718–725, 2017.

30. Kumar, A., Albreem, M. A., Gupta, M., M. Alsharif, M., and Kim, S. "Future 5G network based smart hospitals: Hybrid detection technique for latency improvement", IEEE Access, Vol 8, 153240–153249, 2020.

31. Kumar, A., Gupta, M., Le, D-N., and Aly, A. A. "PTS-PAPR reduction technique for 5g advanced waveforms using BFO algorithm", Intelligent Automation and Soft Computing, Vol 27, No.3, 713–722, 2021.

32. Meena, K., Gupta, M., and Kumar, A. "Analysis of UWB indoor and outdoor channel propagation", IEEE International Women in Engineering (WIE) Conference on Electrical and Computer Engineering (WIECON-ECE), pp. 352–355, 2020.

33. Gupta, M., Chand, L., and Pareek, M. "Power preservation in OFDM using selected mapping (SLM)", Journal of Statistics and Management Systems, Vol.22, No.4, 763–771, 2019.

34. Saeed, M., Hasan, M. K., Hassan, R., Mokhtar, R., Saeed, R.A., Saeid, E., and Gupta, M. "Preserving privacy of user identity based on pseudonym variable in 5G" Computers, Materials & Continua, Vol.70, No.3, 5551–5568, 2022.

35. Adarsh, A., Kumar, B., Gupta, M., Kumar, A., Singh, A., Masud, M., and Alraddady, F. A. "Design of an efficient cooperative spectrum for intra-hospital cognitive radio network" Computers, Materials & Continua, Vol.69, No.1, 35–49, 2021.

36. Kumar, A., Gupta, M., Sharma, M. K., Gupta, M., Chand, L., and Sengar, K. "Role of Detection Techniques in Mobile Communication for Enhancing the Performance of Remote Health Monitoring". In Dinesh Goyal, Shanmugam Balamurugan, Karthikrajan Senthilnathan, Iyswarya Annapoorani, and Mohammad Israr (Eds.), *Cyber-Physical Systems and Industry 4.0*, Apple Academic Press, Chennai, 199–224, 2022.

12 The Role of Terahertz Photoconductive Antennas in Future Healthcare Informatics

Shyamal Mondal, E. Nisha Flora Boby, and
Vaisshale Rathinasamy

CONTENTS

12.1   INTRODUCTION

The frequency of one trillion (10^{12}) cycles per second or 10^{12} Hz can be expressed by the unit 'terahertz'. Terahertz electromagnetic radiation (THz) within the ITU-designated band of frequencies is from 0.3–3 THz (band number 12, Deci millimetric waves) and from 3–30 THz (band number 13, Centimillimetric waves). In recent years, high bandwidth frequencies have been required to have a better wireless communication which led to fifth generation (5G) networks. This demand now leads to sixth generation (6G) using terahertz waves with frequency range from 100 GHz to 10 THz. The wavelength range of THz waves is about 30 μm–3 μm which provides extensive bandwidth resulting in terabits per link with 0.1 bit/sec/Hz being feasible [Elayan, Amin, Shubair, & Alouini (2018)]. So, it became an interesting and challenging field for the researchers to work in this THz-gap. The existence of the THz-gap with the THz being similar to the heatwave, has been noted by two researchers in 1897, H. Rubens and E. F. Nichols. After that, many works have been published in this electromagnetic region under the name of 'far-infrared' or 'sub-millimeter' waves [Blaney (1975); Lamarre, Desert, & Kirchner (1995)]. However, people had no idea about trusted sources and detectors in this region. For the past three decades, it has been gradually understood that THz radiation can contribute to many potential applications [Arnone et al. (1999)]. After the discovery of graphene and carbon nanotubes, researchers have shown that these can also be a good alternative for the generation of THz radiation. A. Geim and K. Novoselov [Geim and Novoselov (2010); Liu et al. (2014)] got the Nobel prize in physics for the use of graphene in different applications including THz generation. There are many challenges in scientific and engineering areas and some of them are also due to the terahertz channels. The THz waves are similar to the RF waves in many aspects, such as directivity, diffraction, and some of the antenna properties. However, the reflectivity, absorption, and transmission through material, especially in the atmosphere, are quite distinct in nature.

The terahertz band has been restricted to some applications due to the lack of efficient terahertz sources and detectors. In recent years, the advancement of terahertz signal generation, detection, communication, and imaging-based applications can be seen [Elayan, Amin, Shihada, Shubair, & Alouini (2019)]. Based on electronic and photonic technology developments, terahertz transceiver design research is advancing day-by-day. The electronic technology to generate the terahertz power has superior advantages in producing the high power while the photonic technologies provide better data rates. The electronic platforms generate THz signals using CMOS technology whereas in the photonic technologies, the photoconductive antennas, quantum cascade lasers, optical down conversion systems and uni-traveling carrier photodiodes support generation beyond 300 GHz frequencies [Kenneth et al. (2019)].

By the integration of hybrid electronic and photonic technology systems, terahertz devices can be designed to have high performance. The high electron mobility, reconfigurable and compact antenna array designs can be attained with plasmonic antennas through the surface plasmon polariton waves in the interface. The signal to noise ratio (SNR) of the THz signal is a very important parameter in the study of biological sample substances. Due to the unavailability of powerful THz sources and detectors, SNR remains low while using THz technology in the medical field. Many research works have been carried out to improve THz sources and to increase the sensitivity of the detectors to obtain high THz SNR. Attenuated total reflection (ATR) spectroscopy is proposed to measure the water content in human skin, but cannot enhance the resonance of target biological substances and is sensitive to few biological samples. Metamaterials can also be used as a sensitive biosensor for the analysis but the frequency range is limited to the metamaterial Fermi level [S.-H. Lee et al. (2020)]. A nano slit with mixed graphene gold electrode can also be used to enhance the terahertz detected signal [Kazemi, Mahani, & Mokhtari (2019)]. Our recent work on interdigitated photoconductive antennas provides a strong terahertz signal which can help to detect biological substances.

12.2 APPLICATIONS OF THZ IN HEALTHCARE SYSTEMS

Recent advancements in terahertz (THz) technology have opened vast THz applications such as THz spectroscopy, imaging, and chemical analysis. The terahertz frequency band has many applications in healthcare and privacy concerns. In the biomedical field, THz spectroscopy has great potential to detect cancer, and for the determination of pathological tissue, and the like. The unique characteristics of terahertz frequencies such as low photon energy, non-ionizing features, and so forth, can be used to assess blood glucose level by monitoring under human skin, hence, it is very useful for diabetic patients in the treatment and prevention of diabetes. Some of the biological samples with various substances like water, proteins, fats, blood, tissue, fiber, vein, and so on, are hard to detect by optical or x-ray imaging but terahertz can detect and distinguish the infected and healthy tissues present in the sample. Blood analysis which is very important in the diagnosis of cancer tumors, can also be achieved through THz imaging and spectroscopy. More than 80% of epithelial tissues are responsible for the growth of several adult cancers, such as lung cancer, skin cancer, breast cancer, colon cancer, liver cancer, bladder cancer, prostate cancer, and so on [Arnone, Ciesla, & Pepper (2000)]. Terahertz radiation can be used to image the human skin for which a penetration depth of a few millimetres is adequate. The biopsies of anomalous skin tissues can be mitigated by the early detection and diagnosis of skin cancers using THz radiation. This is because THz imaging has the ability to distinguish the spectral fingerprints of surface proteins which are the markers for certain cancers. This early-stage detection of cancer using THz analysis reduces the death rate as well as reducing the cost of treatment. By using a THz tomography setup, THz imaging can also be used as a tool to inspect wounds and burns, and to help dentists to detect and diagnose tooth decay and enamel erosion. Currently, X-rays are used for dental imaging which does not help in detecting the early-stage tooth decay [Crawley et al. (2003)]. For medical practitioners, a miniaturized optical fiber-coupled terahertz (THz) endoscope system has been designed to help in diagnosis of various kinds of cancers present in the body [Ji, Lee, Kim, Son, & Jeon (2009)].

12.3 METHODS OF THZ GENERATION

Terahertz science and technology are becoming a popular area in recent research because of the progress both in nanotechnology research and development of high-power lasers. THz waves can be radiated from sources based on either an electronic technique or on optical techniques. Electronic sources rely on RF/MW techniques and optical sources depend purely on optical technologies. Even though the sources in the microwave and infrared frequency bands radiate terahertz with high efficiencies, there are some drawbacks like feasibility, source size, and so forth. Hence to overcome these weaknesses in the techniques, an advanced method of THz sourcing using nano technologies can be used, which is based on a combination of electronic and optical techniques. The sources to generate the terahertz has been discussed in further subsections.

12.3.1 THz Sources Using RF/MW Radiation

Vacuum and solid-state devices are some of the electronic sources that can generate and detect terahertz signals. These sources work based on the principle of electron beam and EMF interactions. There are some other electronic sources such as gyrotron, backward wave-oscillators, and travelling wave tubes that can produce THz frequencies below 1 THz using high-power. Even though they radiate high-power terahertz waves, they are bulky in size and a high magnetic field is required with a high input power. Semiconductor diodes and vacuum tube sources are explained in further subsections, which use electronic techniques to generate the terahertz.

12.3.1.1 Semiconductor Diodes

Diodes like resonant tunnelling diodes (RTD), Gunn diodes, and IMPATT diodes can be used to convert the electronic functionality of the lower frequencies to high frequencies such as the terahertz band. The first terahertz diodes, the whisker contacted devices, are very useful because they are feasible and provide less shunt capacitance. The drawbacks are difficulty in assembly. They have allowed many ground breaking scientific measurements in some applications such as radio astronomy. These semiconductor diodes are based on the negative differential resistance principle. However, these sources have their own advantages and disadvantages. But due to the practical limitations, their performance is degraded dramatically while shifting to higher frequencies. The power from the semiconductor diode is reduced while shifting to higher frequency, because the series resistance increases due to the small size of the diode. Frequency multipliers can also be used to generate terahertz. These are solid-state electronic sources. However, the resultant power of the frequency multiplier is decreased at higher frequencies with limited bandwidth. The doublers and triplers have been implemented in series as the higher order multipliers are inefficient. For example, in series arrangements, the GaAs Schottky diodes can be used as chains of RF/MW sources.

12.3.1.2 Vacuum Tubes

One of the traditional terahertz generation techniques is through microwave tubes which emit free electrons. Some of the THz tube sources are klystron, gyrotron, and travelling wave tube (TWT). In these sources, the electron beam is interacted with the EM waves to generate the THz wave. The source consists of electron gun, regenerative oscillator, depressed collector, and magnetic solenoid which helps in confining the electron beam inside the cavity. Compared to other solid-state components, these tube THz sources produce high powers at lower THz frequencies. These are bulky and larger magnetic bias and voltage power supply is required. To improve the power and efficiency of these devices, special care should be taken on the design of gun, collector, beam transport magnet and the processing circuit.

12.4 THZ SOURCES USING OPTICAL RADIATION

Nonlinear crystals such as ZnTe, LiNbO$_3$, InGaAs, GaP, and the like, are very common terahertz sources that exploit the nonlinear optical properties by optical rectification (OR) and difference frequency generation (DFG) methods when illuminated by ultrashort laser pulses. Semiconductor materials like germanium, silicon, and the like, can also be used to build the THz laser source. Under the condition of semiconductor defected structure, the lasers rely on the population inversion. These lasers provide a better tunability over a wide range of wavelengths. The two down conversion processes, such as, difference frequency generation (DFG) and optical rectification (OR) can be used to generate the coherent terahertz waves with high spectral resolution. A wide terahertz bandwidth can be obtained using these nonlinear processes. The coherent and tunable THz waves can be generated using organic nonlinear crystal, such as, DAST (4-N, N-dimethylamino-4'-N'-methyl-stilbazolium tosylate), DSTMS (4-N, N-dimethylamino-4'-N'-methyl-stilbazolium 2,4,6-trimethylbenzenesulfonate), and so forth. The THz waves can also be efficiently achieved using an annealed ZnGeP$_2$ crystal based on the DFG phase matching configuration. The phase matching between the THz and the optical fields is one of its major limitations. Moreover, the thickness of the nonlinear material should be carefully chosen, and high optical power is required to generate high terahertz power.

12.4.1 Lasers

Terahertz radiation can be generated directly from various lasers, such as, molecular lasers, semiconductor lasers, and the like. A few tens of milliwatts of THz power is produced from the low-pressure flowing gas cavities, while injecting a grating tuned CO$_2$ laser. In the near-IR and visible frequency range, the semiconductor diode lasers are predominantly used with appropriate bandgap materials. The quantum-cascade laser (QCL) can also be used to generate terahertz waves. QCL is a unipolar semiconductor laser which operates differently from other semiconductor diodes and generates THz radiation between 2–5 THz. To have the lasing condition in QCL, the population inversion condition must be satisfied. To achieve this, the thickness of semiconductor layers and bias voltage should be considered carefully. The energy of the system can be improved by reducing the thickness of the semiconductor. A pulsed and continuous wave terahertz is generated using the QCL and the operating frequency is based on the quantum well design. Stable and reliable terahertz photons are generated directly from QCL with high output power. The main drawback of QCL is that it can be operated only under cryogenic temperature [Fathololoumi et al. (2012)].

12.4.2 PLASMA

THz generation can be obtained from laser-induced plasma while the high peak power pulsed laser beam is focusing in air or any inert gaseous medium. The simplest process for plasma generation is to focus two separate wavelengths simultaneously in a nonlinear medium to have two color plasma which leads to the terahertz generation. The illuminated laser beam has sufficient intensity to trigger the plasma filament through higher order nonlinear frequency mixing processes. As a result, any two nearby frequencies with high electric field beating each other leads to broadband THz radiation [Kim (2009)]. For example, the ultrafast Ti:Sapphire laser pulses with 100 fs pulse width and 1 mJ pulse energy are sufficient to create THz-plasma radiation.

12.5 THZ SOURCES COMBINING OPTICAL, ELECTRONIC AND MAGNETIC FIELDS

THz generation and detection is also possible when the electronic properties of semiconductors are exploited in the presence of optical fields. Based on the principle of photoconductivity in the semiconductor materials, these sources are created. In the source, over the semiconductor material, a voltage-based antenna is printed. The ultrashort femtosecond laser pulse is used for excitation and photocarrier generation in the material. Based on optical excitation, the terahertz sources are divided into continuous-wave THz sources and pulsed THz sources.

12.5.1 SPINTRONICS MATERIALS

There are three generations of spintronic devices as follows: based on spin transport and the spin dynamics employing electric field, based of spin–orbit effects and electromagnetic coupling, and using three-dimensional structures and quantum engineering. The ferromagnetic metal layer sandwiched between two non-magnetic metal layers is used as a THz source where the spin current in the magnetic layer leads to THz generation. Later, the generated THz waves is diffused through the non-magnetic part of the device using a super-diffusive process. The advantages of spintronic emitters are that they are easy-to-use, robust, efficient, and don't require any electrical connections. These types of spintronic materials can be fabricated through lithographic techniques.

12.5.2 PHOTO MIXERS

Terahertz generation from photo mixers can be obtained using two CW lasers having frequencies very close to each other. The schematic of the photo mixer to generate the terahertz wave is represented in Figure 12.1. Two single mode lasers, with

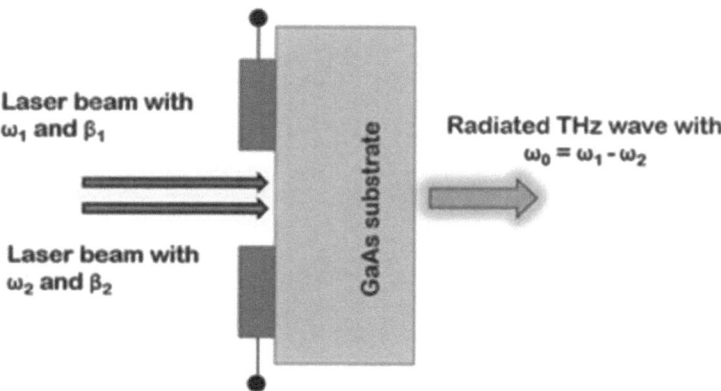

FIGURE 12.1 Schematic diagram of terahertz photo mixer.

frequencies of ω_1 and ω_2 and phases of β_1 and β_2 respectively, are merged using a beam combiner and propagate collinearly. The resulting beam is targeted on the DC-biased THz photo mixer antenna to generate THz radiation of ω_0 frequency (where, $\omega_0 = \omega_1 - \omega_2$) (see Figure 12.2). The optical frequencies of the CW-laser beams can be varied by tuning the laser cavity length, the optical grating structures, and the operating temperature. The optical sources used for photo mixers are generally the laser diodes, and the system is compact in structure with less complexity and light weight. The geometry of the photo mixer also affects the photocurrent and optical to terahertz conversion efficiencies. The dipole photo mixer gives high carrier density, high photocurrent, and better conversion efficiencies. But in this geometry, the electric field distribution is not uniform. Hence, to attain a uniform electric field distribution, interdigitated-like structures can be incorporated. This geometry has higher conductance as well as higher gap capacitance between the electrodes which helps to generate a high THz electric field. Moreover, it has much less screening effect compared to the dipole PCA.

12.5.3 THE PHOTOCONDUCTIVE ANTENNA

Photoconductive antennas (PCA) are made of semiconductor substrate material with the metal electrodes placed on the top of the substrate, a laser source, and a DC bias voltage. In earlier literature, they are referred to as Auston switches as they were first discovered by Auston in 1984, similar to the Hertzian dipole structure. The THz PCA works with the principle of photoconduction. An ultrashort laser pulse with photon energy higher than the photoconductive material bandgap is excited on the THz PCA. The photocarriers are created and then bias voltage is applied to the electrodes. The photocarriers are accelerated towards the corresponding electrodes by the biased electric field and generate the photocurrent which drives the antenna to radiate the terahertz waves as represented in Figure 12.2. To generate the pulsed THz system, the PCA can be used both as an emitter and detector which is based on the ultra-fast optical techniques.

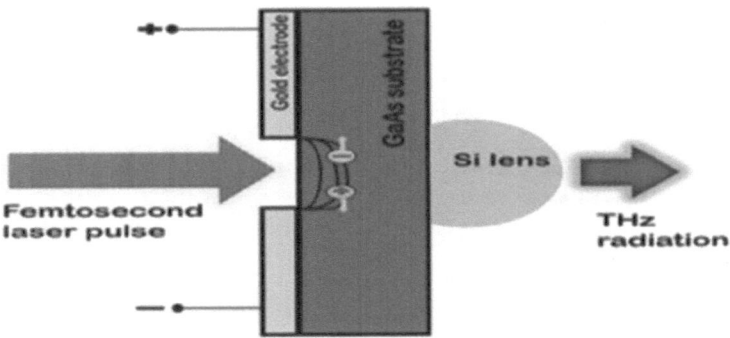

FIGURE 12.2   Biased THz emitter PCA.

In RF/MW antennas, the substrate material should be a low loss dielectric material, such as fiberglass-reinforced-epoxy-laminate sheet. Gallium arsenide (GaAs) having high carrier mobility can be used as the substrate material in the monolithic micro-wave integrated circuit (MMIC). But in THz PCA, semiconductor materials like silicon, GaAs, InGaAs and low temperature grown-GaAs (LT-GaAs) can be used because of their characteristics, such as high electron mobility, supporting high bias voltage, ultra-short carrier lifetime, and high intrinsic resistivity. Metals such as gold, silver, aluminium, and the like, can be used for biasing pads as well as antenna electrodes. The advantages of PCAs are that it is simple, compact, capable of gener-ating moderate THz intensity without pumping by a high-power laser source and that it operates at room temperature.

12.6   IMPORTANCE OF PCA

In the previous section, the advantages and drawbacks of various THz sources have been discussed. Among these sources, the photoconductive antenna shows better per-formance in different aspects of THz generation [Ferguson & Zhang (2002)]. It can be easily integrated in fiber optics laser systems. Hence, it can be operated remotely in outdoor conditions. Therefore, in many applications, such as, medical diagnostics, agro applications, defense and security applications, manufacturing industries and many more, these PCAs are highly acceptable.

12.7   CLASSIFICATIONS OF PCA

Based on the antenna gap size, the terahertz PCAs are generally classified into small gap antennas, semi-large gap antennas, and large gap antennas. There are different types of antenna structures. some of these are dipole, bowtie, interdigitated structures, nano-antennas, split ring resonators, and so forth. These different antenna structures can be optimized to provide better performance in THz radiation. The performance of PCA depends on the optical source, geometrical parameters, and antenna impedance matching. The geometry considerations for the antenna electrode is more important as the photocarriers are created in the active area. The geometry of the antenna also affects the mobility as well as the generation rate of the photocarriers which depends on the electric field distribution. To enhance the radiated THz power, antenna electrodes with sharp edges can be used that can operate with even less input optical power. Even-though the edge of the electrodes is very important to get high electric-field, the fabrication of sharp tiny edge antenna electrodes is difficult. Screening effects, velocity overshoot phenomenon, and the like, are some of the restriction phenomena in the generation of terahertz photocurrent [Cai et al. (1997)].

12.7.1 DIPOLE PCA

The first Hertzian dipole antenna similar to a photoconductive switch has been used both as a terahertz emitter and detector, proposed by Auston et al. [Auston, Cheung, & Smith (1984)]. The dipole geometry as shown in Figure 12.3 is the simplest design of PCA for THz radiation and it is being used because of its simplicity in design, and because it is less complex in nature. The electrodes can be biased using contact pads, coplanar strip line, and so forth, to accelerate the generated photocarriers towards their respective electrodes. Factors such as photoconduction, the duration of optical pulses, and the geometry of PCA affects the radiated power, efficiency, bandwidth, and sensitivity for the terahertz radiation. But this dipole structured PCA has a larger gap between the two electrodes, so the carrier drifting time is increased. Only a few photocarriers reach their corresponding electrodes and the remaining pairs end up in recombination as a result of the screening effect which leads to a reduction of terahertz radiation. So, to mitigate this effect and to boost PCA performance, the antenna geometry has to be modified with small antenna gap within the active area.

12.7.2 BOWTIE PCA

To radiate terahertz, a bow-tie antenna which is printed on a semiconductor photo-conductive substrate can be used which is similar to the dipole PCA. This bow-tie shaped antenna as shown in Figure 12.4 is the first introduced standard design as

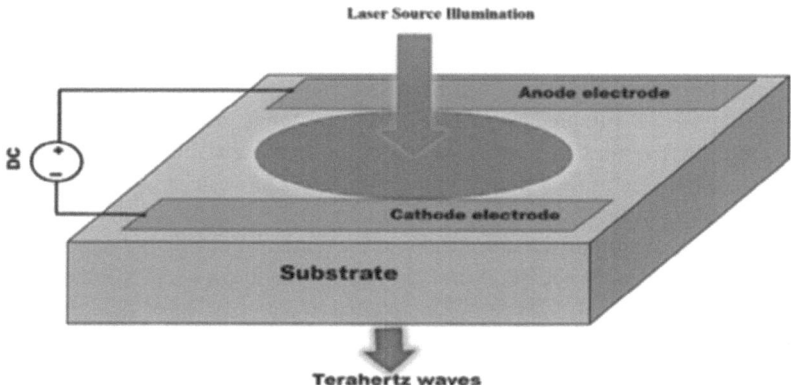

FIGURE 12.3   Structure of dipole PCA.

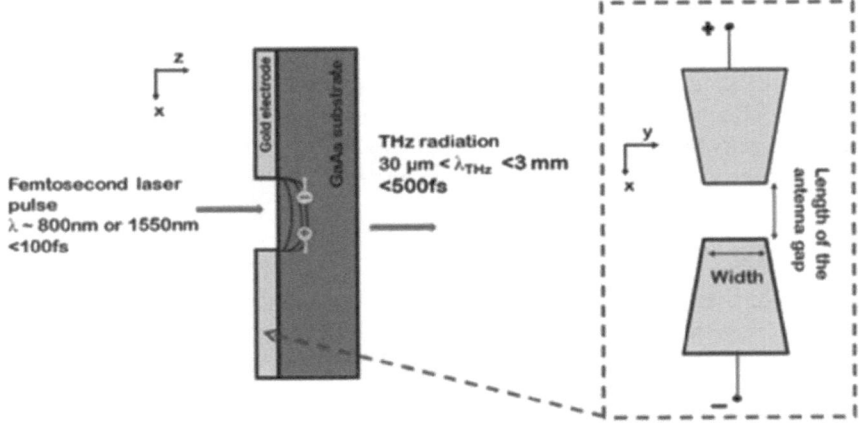

FIGURE 12.4 Bow-tie photoconductive antenna.

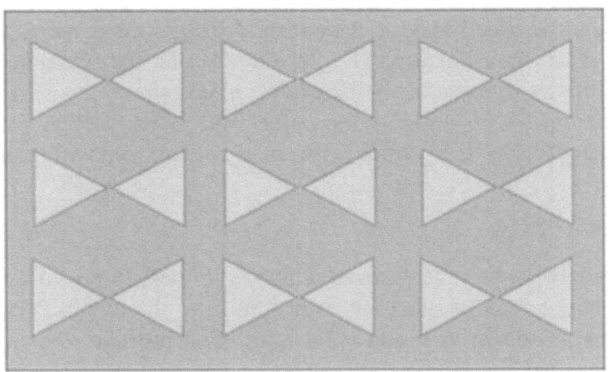

FIGURE 12.5 Bow-tie photoconductive antenna array.

a photoconductive emitter and acts as an appropriate reference case. The DC bias voltage is applied across the arms of the bow-tie antenna. As mentioned for the dipole PCA, the transient photocurrent is generated in the bowtie PCA by the acceleration of carriers, resulting in the terahertz emission. With motivation from the design (see Figure 12.4) in [Khiabani, Huang, Shen, & Boyes (2013)], many innovative designs are proposed to overcome the drawbacks of the general PCA performance. This bow-tie element is integrated with an artificial magnetic conductor (AMC) or a silicon lens to reinforce its directivity. The bow-tie antenna array can also be designed as shown in Figure 12.5 by connecting the DC bias and ground lines in series to their respective electrodes. One capacitance can be employed parallel to the DC source to nullify the fluctuations in DC source. The bow-tie shaped antenna consists of aluminium, titanium, silver, gold, metal films in some micrometer thicknesses over a substrate material such as LT-GaAs, SI-GaAs, and the like. Each electrode of the bowtie looks like a trapezoid in which the width of the small arm and large arm can be increased so that the resonant frequency can be varied. To tune the antenna at an operating frequency, the width of the antenna should be properly selected. The radiation efficiency is far improved while using the silicon lens based bowtie PCA.

12.7.3 INTERDIGITATED PCA

To emit the terahertz field with large spectral bandwidth and with high SNR, innovative antenna geometry designs, are proposed which help in the terahertz research area. The 3D schematic diagram of the interdigitated PCA electrode structure is given in Figure 12.6. The interdigitated photoconductive antenna (IPCA) geometry helps in overcoming the drawbacks of other antenna designs. There are interdigitated photo mixers for continuous THz radiation and interdigitated photoconductive antennas to emit the pulsed terahertz. In this structure, finger like electrodes are added to the photoconductive active area gap (like dipole PCA) on the top of semiconductor substrate material.

The large gap and small gap antenna have their own pros and cons. The IPCAs combine the advantages of both large aperture and small aperture antennas. The advantages of having a large area between the dipole electrodes are high carrier density, high power, less laser repetition rate, reduction of diffraction and the fact that the use of a silicon lens can be avoided. But due to the large gap, many unpaired carriers cause a screening effect which affects the PCA performance. This can be mitigated by placing inter-weaved fingers in the antenna gap area which reduces the gap between the electrodes and also reduces the carrier drift time. Because of this small gap due to the placement of interdigitated electrodes, the antenna is driven with less input power and leads to high terahertz electric fields, high SNR compared to the large gap antennas such as dipoles, bow-tie antennas, and the like. To make the

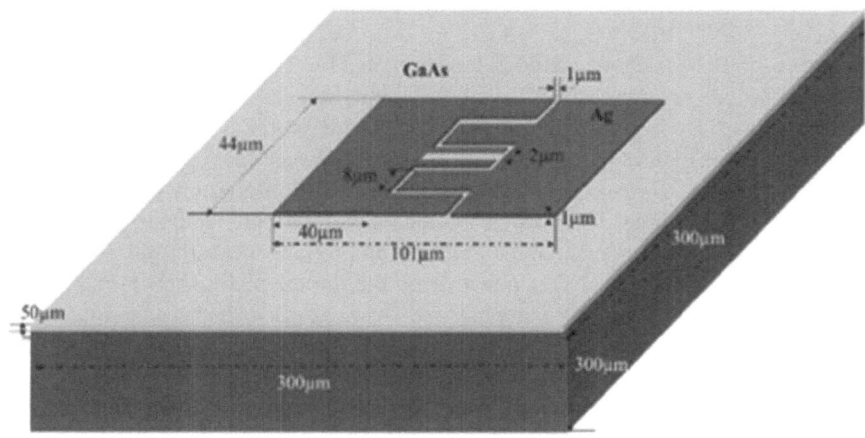

FIGURE 12.6   Schematic diagram of slot IPCA 3D view.

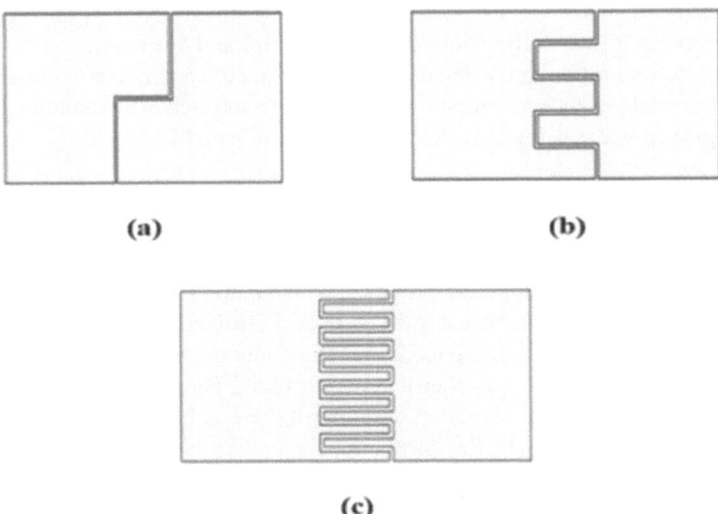

(a)   (b)

(c)

FIGURE 12.7   Top view of (a) 2-elements interdigitated PCA (b) 5-elements interdigitated PCA (c) 13-elements interdigitated PCA.

electric field distribution uniform and to accelerate the carriers, several techniques, such as having a second metallization layer, binary phase masking, a micro lens array, can be employed in the interdigitated structures. This leads to further improvement in the optical to terahertz conversion efficiency. The number of elements in the IPCA can be varied (such as, 2 elements, 5 elements, 14 elements) as shown in Figure 12.7, by keeping the area and gap constant, to increase the efficiency of PCA [Rathinasamy, Thipparaju, Edwin, & Monda (2021); Rathinasamy, Thipparaju, Boby, & Mondal (2022)].

12.7.3.1   Tip-to-Tip PCA

The tip-to-tip PCA is another kind of interdigitated PCA where the cathode and anode electrode fingers are distributed like a comb structure, and they meet head-to-head at the central gap. By introducing this tip-to-tip geometry, the electric field distribution is stronger in the central part of PCA where the fingers are placed in a horizontal position. There are also tip-to-tip trapezoidal fingers which produce two-fold stronger electric field magnitude. The bow-tie antenna along with the rectangular tip-to-tip or trapezoidal tip-to-tip fingers can also be used to produce terahertz pulses [Khiabani, et al. (2013)]. The detected THz power from the trapezoidal tip-to-tip PCA is seven times more than the bare gap antennas and twice as good as the rectangular tip-to-tip geometries [Khiabani, et al. (2013)]. The geometry of rectangular tip to tip and trapezoidal tip to tip interdigitated PCA is given in Figure 12.8(a) and Figure 12.8(b) respectively. The trapezoidal tip-to-tip structure represented in Figure 12.8(b) produces 1.37 µW power and the interdigitated PCA produces 0.68 µW power whilst the dipole PCA produces 0.19 µW power at 0.17 THz frequency. The trapezoidal tip

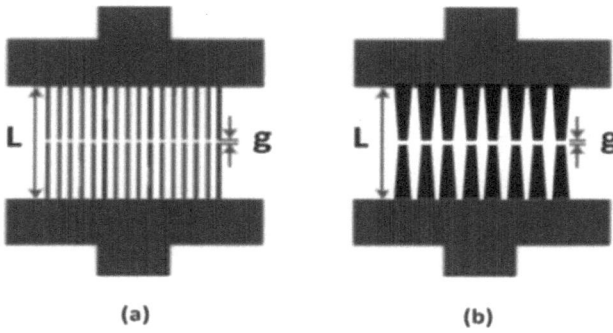

FIGURE 12.8   Different shapes of tip-to-tip interdigitated electrode: (a) Rectangular (b) Trapezoidal.

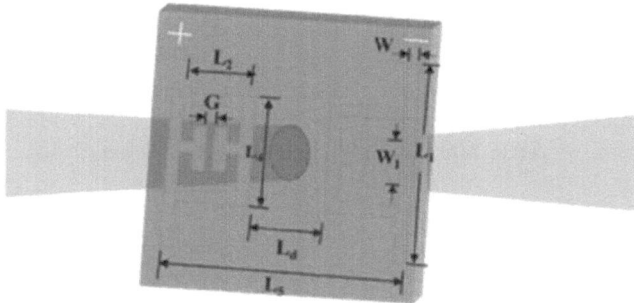

FIGURE 12.9   Structural diagram of split ring resonator.

to tip IPCA can produce high electric-field compared to the rectangular tip to tip and dipole PCA.

12.7.4   Split Ring Resonator PCA

designed in the shape of a split ring resonator (SRR). The structure of the SRR is shown in Figure 12.9. The resonant behaviour of the photo-induced current is due to the inductance nature of the SRR electrode structure based on the lumped circuit model. The current flow is induced between the cathode and anode of the SRR PCA by laser illumination which in turn leads to the THz generation. This variation in current becomes the source of radiation of THz electromagnetic waves. The generated THz field and the photocurrent is described by the Equation 12.1 [K. Lee et al. (2020)].

$$E_{THz} \, \alpha \, \frac{dI(t)}{dt} \qquad (12.1)$$

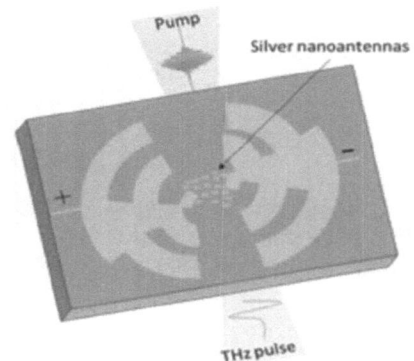

FIGURE 12.10   Illustration of the silver nano-antennas in the gap of log-periodic PCA.

The incident plane wave is perpendicular to the SRR surface, and the electric field excites the electro-magnetic modes (EM modes) of the SRR. The structure is symmetrical, and the equivalent circuit consists of two inductors and one capacitor. The inductance value depends on the whole electrode length (L_4) and width (L_2) whereas the capacitance of the SRR depends on the gap width G and length W_1.

12.7.5 NANO-STRUCTURED PCA

To improve the optical to terahertz conversion efficiency, researchers are inclined towards nano-antennas, nano-structured arrays, double layer nano-plasmonic structures, nano-rods, and the like. The screening effect, the low absorption coefficient and lower quantum efficiency are vital factors which affect PCA performance. To overcome these phenomena, nano-structured antennas can be used. In the last few years, the plasmonic effect couples the EM field with surface electrons to enhance electric field distribution as well as the absorption coefficient and also improves the efficiency of PCA. This is also known as hybrid THz-optical PCA. The silver nano-antennas in the active area of the log-periodic antenna are shown in Figure 12.10. The experimental results of nano-antenna based PCAs generate better output power compared to the conventional PCA [Lepeshov, et al. (2017)]. For photonics and optoelectronic devices, such as, photodetectors, optical modulators, optical filters, photo mixers, photoconductive antennas, the plasmonic effect can be involved where the device dimensions are comparable to the operating wavelength. Han Sang-Pil, et al. [Han et al. (2011)] proposed a gold nano-island array in the antenna gap between the electrodes to improve the photocurrent and absorption coefficient of THz PCA.

12.8 METHODS OF THZ DETECTION

The growth of the THz detection devices over time is faster than the growth of the THz generation devices. The issue in detecting the terahertz is the photon energy of 0.41–41 meV at this THz frequency region [Khiabani (2013)]. The THz energy is very

close to the background thermal noise energy, whereas it can be mitigated by cryogenic cooling. Coherent detection techniques can be used to determine the amplitude
and phase of the received signal however when using the incoherent technique, only
intensity can be measured. Both narrowband and broadband signals can be detected
using terahertz detectors. Heterodyne circuits, electro-optic sampling technique and
THz PCA can be used in the coherent type of detection to detect the terahertz signal.
In the incoherent detection, lenses and mirrors are always used to focus and guide
the THz beam onto the detector. The unwanted signals can be removed from the
THz signal through a coherent detection process. Some of the direct THz power
measurement detectors where phase cannot be measured, are Golay cells, pyroelec-
tric detectors, and bolometers, which can be used at room temperature. For a lower
response time, the THz can be measured by a cryogenically cooled semiconductor
detector.

12.8.1 ELECTRO-OPTIC SAMPLING METHOD

Electro-optic sampling is also known as Pockels effect in nonlinear crystals.
Figure 12.11. shows a representation of the electro-optic sampling method. The
polarization rotation of the optical beam is detected by the balanced photodiode in
the presence of the THz beam in the electro-optic (and nonlinear crystal) medium.
The terahertz pulse from the emitter and the probe laser pulse (split from the beam
splitter) passes collinearly into an electro-optic crystal. This incoming THz signal
electric field is directly proportional to the birefringence (generated by the Pockels
effect) of the EO crystals. The first order electro-optic effect rotates the polarization
of the optical probe beam. This change in polarization is accounted for by a balanced
detector placed behind a quarter wave plate (QWP) and a Wollaston prism. The QWP
converts the linear polarization into a circular or elliptical polarization depending
on the amplitude of the electric field components. The Wollaston prism/polariza-
tion sensitive beam splitter separates two orthogonal polarizations into two identical

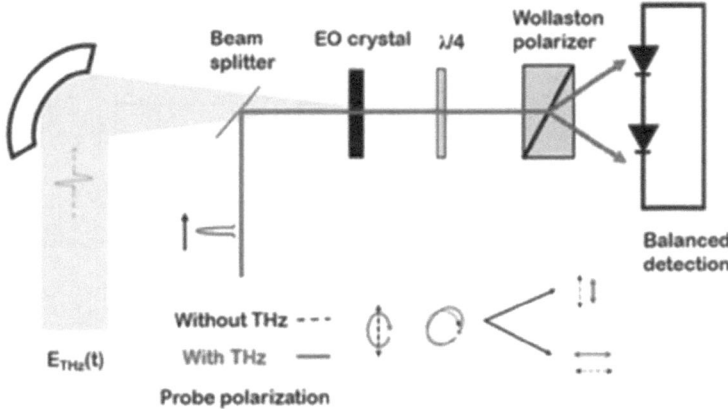

FIGURE 12.11   Illustration of electro-optic sampling.

photodetectors. The difference between both photodetector signals determines the magnitude and phase of the THz signal. The higher the incoming THz signal at the EO crystal, the greater is the difference in the signal at the balanced photodetectors. This process can detect the phase of the THz signal as the optical pulse (~ 10s of *fs* order) which is much shorter than the THz pulse (~ *ps* order) while sampling it. This electro-optic sampling method is very sensitive to environmental noise, therefore, the measurement of the balanced photodiode signal through a lock-in amplifier is absolutely necessary to achieve a noiseless detection.

12.8.2 THz Heterodyne Detector

To detect the weak and narrowband signals, a coherent detection technique such as heterodyne detection can also be used. The block diagram of a heterodyne detector to detect emitted terahertz waves is given in Figure 12.12. Nonlinear devices such as the Schottky diode, tunnel diodes, and bolometers are used in the mixers to combine the terahertz signal with the local signal. The high frequency signals are then filtered out and by maintaining the amplitude and phase, the intermediate frequency (IF) remains at the output. This down conversion of the terahertz signal to the IF frequency is the coherent heterodyne detection. This detector can be employed for high sensitivity applications in cryogenic temperatures.

12.8.3 THz PCA

To detect the terahertz signal, a photoconductive antenna is a good choice. The working principle of the THz PCA detector is the same as the PCA emitter except for the biasing. The incoming signal electric field creates a voltage which causes the carriers to accelerate. The photocurrent detected with a time delay of *t* can be explained using Equation 12.2,

$$J_{det} = E_{THz}(t) * \sigma_{det}(t) \tag{12.2}$$

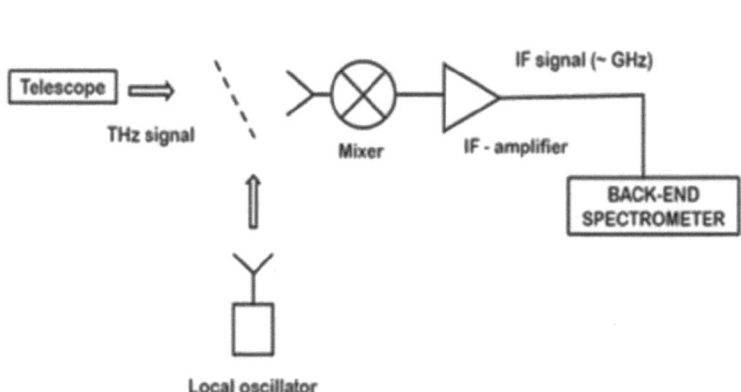

FIGURE 12.12   THz heterodyne detection technique.

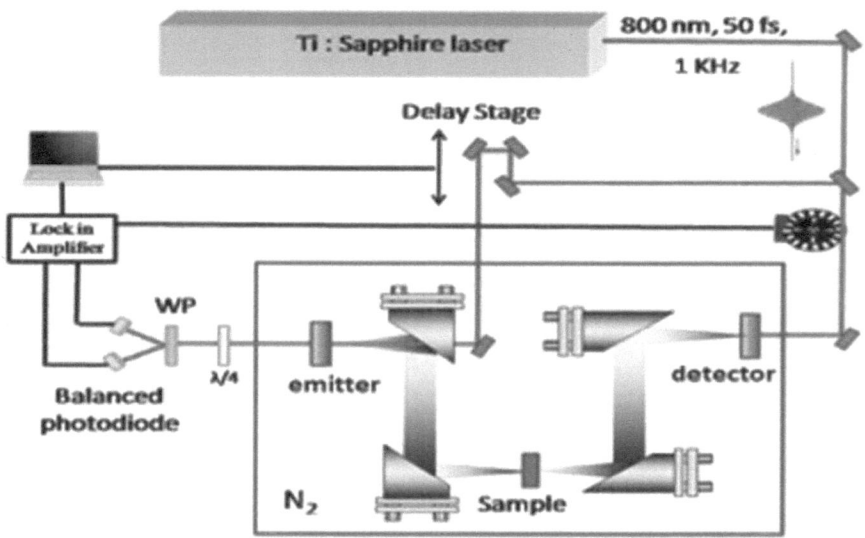

FIGURE 12.13   Schematic diagram of experimental setup for THz generation and detection.

The arrival time of the pulse is adjusted by the variable time delay and the THz photocurrent is measured using the ammeter. The photoconductive antenna on the detector side acts as a low pass filter. The experimental setup (THz time domain spectroscopy, THz-TDS) used for the generation and detection of THz-pulsed radiation is shown in Figure 12.13. In this setup, the photoconductive antenna is used as an emitter and also as a detector. The ultrashort laser source of 800 nm wavelength with 1 kHz repetition rate and pulse duration of 50 fs from the Kerr-lens mode locked Ti:Sapphire laser amplifier is used as the optical input source. Parabolic mirrors are used to focus the generated terahertz beam into the sample. Then, another two parabolic mirrors are used to collimate and focus the detected beam on the detector. A delay is introduced between the optical pulse and terahertz pulse using a motorized delay stage (MDS). At the THz receiver, an optical probe beam is creating the excited photocarriers which are accelerated by the time dependent electric field components of the incoming THz signal. The noise-free data-acquisition is obtained through a lock-in amplifier. It is to be noted that a PCA based THz receiver is always connected to an amplifier circuit. The THz detection using PCA is simple and reliable than other coherent detection techniques.

12.9   EQUIVALENT CIRCUITAL ANALYSIS OF PCA

The working principle of PCA can be described through an electrical model using an equivalent circuit. The femtosecond laser beam is illuminated on the gap area between the electrodes. The photocarriers are created only if the incident photon energy is higher than the semiconductor band gap energy. Then the applied DC bias voltage

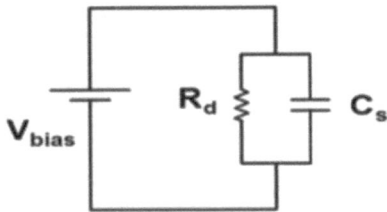

FIGURE 12.14   Dipole PCA equivalent circuit in dark state.

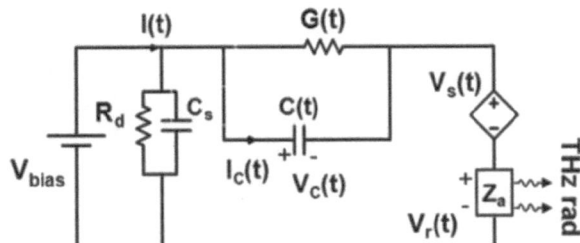

FIGURE 12.15   Dipole PCA equivalent circuit with combined dark state and illuminated state.

creates an electric field distribution and accelerates the electron-hole pair towards the corresponding electrodes which leads to the generation of a photocurrent. The terahertz is radiated from the antenna by the rate of change of this photocurrent. The left-over carrier without reaching the electrodes leads to the screening effect which is predicted by the equivalent circuit. As the electrode gap dimensions are less than the radiated wavelength, we can apply the lumped element approach along with the carrier dynamics to model the equivalent circuit. The dark resistance R_d and capacitance C_s is due to the flow of dark current in semiconductor substrate material without laser illumination [Krotkus et al. (1995)] which is shown in Figure 12.14. Figure 12.15 represents the equivalent circuit of the dipole PCA by combining both the dark state and the optical illuminated state. The gap conductance ($G(t)$) and the gap capacitance ($C(t)$) is created when the antenna is optically illuminated, and it represents the generation of plasma in the antenna active region. The antenna impedance (Z_a) is used to determine the power loss during the antenna radiation [Gregory et al. (2003)]. The screening voltage, capacitance voltage, and the conductance of the PCA are time dependent. To improve the performance of PCA and to extract the analytical relation between the time-dependent parameters, researchers are working on the interdigitated PCA structure simulation and its theoretical analysis through the equivalent circuit model. In the IPCA design, the cathode and anode finger-like structures in the gap area are parallel to each other [Godyak, Piejak, & Alexandrovich (1991)]. Hence, the number of parallel combinations of gap capacitance ($C(t)$) and conductance ($G(t)$) depends on the number of interdigitated structures. By applying Kirchhoff's law to the equivalent circuit, the time dependent radiation voltage ($V_r(t)$), capacitance voltage ($V_c(t)$) and screening voltage ($V_s(t)$) can be calculated and analysed using the Drude-Lorentz model (explained in the next section), the energy balanced transport model [Emadi, Safian, & Nezhad (2017)], the drift diffusion model [Prajapati, Bharadwaj, Chatterjee, & Bhattacharjee (2017); Boby, Prajapati, Rathinasamy, Rao, & Mondal (2022)], and so forth.

12.10 NUMERICAL SIMULATIONS OF PCA

The simulation of PCAs is always required before an experimental investigation. It can be performed by using commercial software, such as, Silvaco/Sentaurus TCAD, Ansys HFSS, CST Microwave Studio Suite, or COMSOL Multiphysics package. The drift diffusion model is used to determine the density of carriers in the active layer of the substrate. The contribution of holes is not considered in the calculation because of their high mass and less mobility compared to the electrons. The carrier density is directly proportional to the optical generation rate, and it increases with a decrease in the carrier lifetime. The time dependent carrier density is calculated by using the continuity equation as Equation 12.3

$$\frac{dn(t)}{dt} = -\frac{n(t)}{\tau_c} + g(t) \tag{12.3}$$

where, $n(t)$ is the carrier density, τ_c is the carrier lifetime and $g(t)$ is the photocarrier generation-rate. The optical source is considered as a Gaussian laser beam. The carrier-generation rate by the laser in a PCA is given in Equation 12.4

$$g(t) = \frac{2\eta P(t)}{\pi \omega_0^2 h v_{opt} V} \tag{12.4}$$

where, η is the quantum efficiency, $P(t)$ is the optical power, ω_0 is the beam waist radius, h is Planck's constant v_{opt} is the laser frequency, V is the active volume. The quantum efficiency η, the generation of photocarriers inside the semiconductor, can be defined as in Equation 12.5

$$\eta = (1 - R_{coeff})\left[1 - exp(-\alpha T_{LT-GaAs})\right] \qquad 12.5$$

Where, R_{coeff} is the power reflection coefficient, α is the optical absorption coefficient, $T_{LT-GaAs}$ is the skin depth. The optical power within the laser beam having pulse duration (τ_l) and beam waist radius (ω_0) is described in Equation 12.6

$$P(t) = P_0\left[1 - exp\left(\frac{-2r^2}{\omega_0^2}\right)\right]exp\left(\frac{-2t^2}{\tau_l^2}\right) \tag{12.6}$$

where, P_0 is the optical peak power. The average carrier density can be calculated using Equation 12.7

$$n_{avg}(t) = \frac{A.n(t)}{V_a} \tag{12.7}$$

In dipole PCA, the total area where the carriers are generated is given as, area, $A = L_d W_d$ and the active volume is given as, volume, $V_a = L_d W_d T_{LT\text{-}GaAs}$. Where, L_d and W_d are the length and width of the active area respectively. While adding interdigitated fingers in the active area at the bare gap of dipole PCA, the carriers are generated in the gap between the fingers. The area of the interdigitated gap should be considered in the calculation of the IPCA structure. To know about the conduction of current across the antenna gap, the conductance can be evaluated as given in Equation 12.8 [Prajapati et al. (2017)]

$$G(t) = q\mu_e n(t)\left(\frac{W_d}{L_d}\right)T_{LT-GaAs} \tag{12.8}$$

where, $n(t)$ is the carrier density, μ_e is the mobility of electrons, q is the charge of an electron. Due to the polarization of charges, the screening effect arises, which should be reduced to increase the THz photocurrent [El-Ghazaly, Joshi, & Grondin (1990)]. The $V_c(t)$ can be calculated using the radiated voltage and the screening voltage and it is written as Equation 12.9

$$V_c(t) = V_{bias} - V_r(t) - V_s(t) \tag{12.9}$$

where, $V_c(t)$ is the gap capacitance voltage, $V_{bias}(t)$ is the applied bias voltage, $V_r(t)$ is the radiating voltage, $V_s(t)$ is the screening voltage. The screening voltage can be calculated as Equation 12.10 [Prajapati et al. (2017)], [Khiabani et al. (2013)],

$$V_s(t) = \beta(t)V_c(t) \tag{12.10}$$

where, $\beta(t)$ is the screening voltage coefficient [Khiabani et al. (2013)]. The radiated voltage can be calculated by using Equation 12.11

$$V_r(t) = G(t)V_c(t)Z_a + I_c(t)Z_a \tag{12.11}$$

where, Z_a is the antenna impedance, I_c is the time dependent capacitance current. The capacitor current is given in Equation 12.12

$$I_c(t) = \frac{\pi q\mu_e^2 \Delta t W_e n(t)V_c^2(t)}{4L_{gap}^2} \tag{12.12}$$

where, Δt is the time step. The total current flowing through the circuit can be written as Equation 12.13

$$I_{total}(t) = G(t)V_c(t) + I_c(t) + \frac{V_{bias}}{R_d} \tag{12.13}$$

where, $I_{total}(t)$ is the total current, R_d is the dark resistance. The THz photocurrent generated by the laser illumination on the semiconductor material is calculated numerically by solving Equation 12.13. The terahertz radiated power can be calculated in Equation 12.14

$$P_{THz}(t) = I_{total}(t)^2 Z_a \qquad (12.14)$$

There are three types of efficiencies for PCA, such as, optical to electrical conversion efficiency η_e, THz radiation efficiency η_r and matching efficiency η_m. The overall efficiency is expressed in Equation 12.15

$$\eta_t = \frac{P_{THz}(peak)}{P_{opt}} \qquad (12.15)$$

where, P_{opt} is the optical input power and $P_{THz}(peak)$ is the peak terahertz radiated power. This total efficiency can be increased by increasing the η_e, as it is the ratio of electrical power to optical power. The normalized electric field for the interdigitated photoconductive antenna design is obtained by increasing the number of interdigitated elements. Figure 12.16(a) shows the simulated results for the IPCA structure given in Figure 12.6. The frequency roll-off and ripples increase based on the number

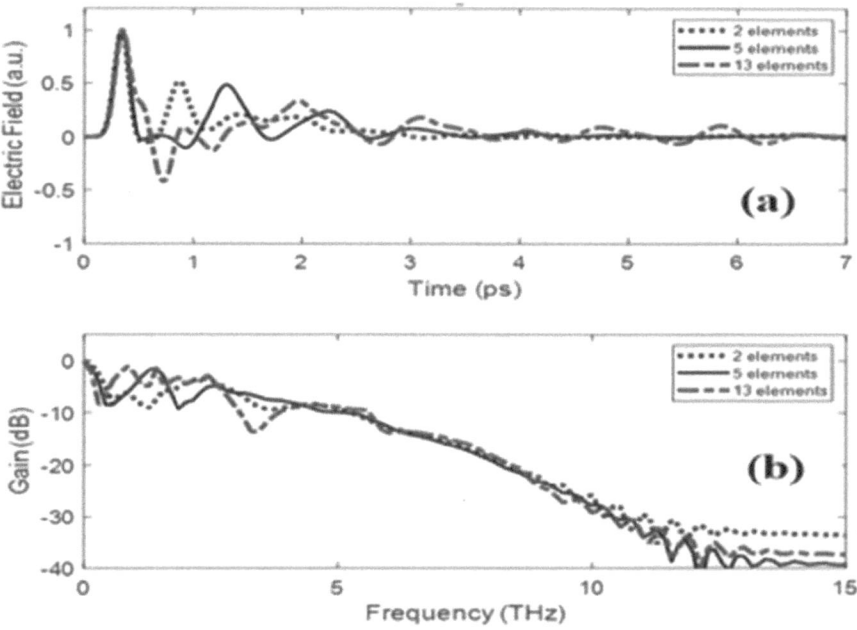

FIGURE 12.16 (a) Simulated E-field for the IPCA and (b) Gain for the different elements of IPCA.

of elements. Figure 12.16(b) depicts the frequency spectrum which clearly shows the ripples for the 2-interdigitated elements, 5-interdigitated elements and 13-interdigitated elements. Hence, this briefs us to design the antenna with various numbers of elements to achieve broadband to narrow band applications [Boby, Prajapati, Rathinasamy, Mukherjee, & Mondal (2022)].

12.11   EXPERIMENTAL ANALYSIS THROUGH THZ SPECTROSCOPY AND IMAGING

THz science with existing technologies has achieved a remarkable progress in medical diagnostics experimentally. The early detection and diagnosis of several diseases can be achieved using THz spectroscopy and imaging techniques. Among many possibilities, two of the techniques of blood sugar measurement and tumor-cancer detection are described below.

12.11.1   A Non-invasive Blood Sugar Measurement Method

Non-invasive blood sugar measurement is possible using a THz time domain spectroscopic technique through which diabetes can be diagnosed. In this investigation, sub-THz radiation (around 0.1 THz) has been used because of its lower absorption of water in glucose solution. The concentration of glucose in the blood can be identified using reflectance measurement for measuring the blood glucose through this non-invasive technique.

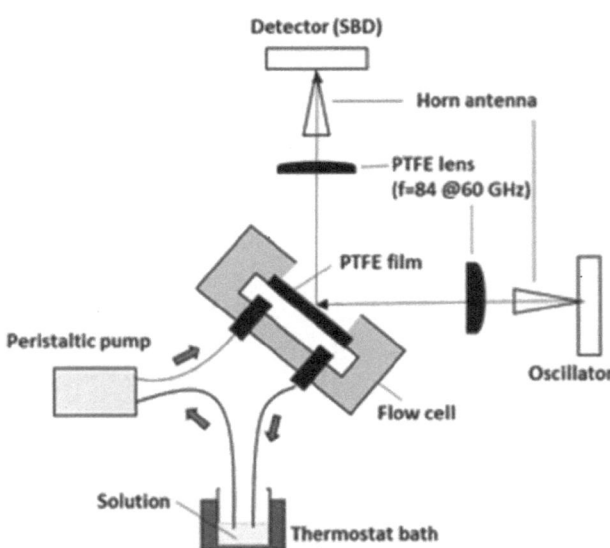

FIGURE 12.17   Schematic diagram of the optical configuration showing the sub-THz reflection measurement system for measuring the glucose in blood using a non-invasive technique.

Figure 12.17 shows the schematic diagram of the optical configuration showing the sub-THz reflection measurement system for measuring the glucose in blood using a non-invasive technique. The semiconductor oscillator device emits THz radiation which is focused by a polytetrafluoroethylene (PTFE) lens to the flow cell. The blood sample is circulated onto the flow cell using a peristaltic pump. Hence, another PTFE lens focuses the THz beam after reflection from the flow cell. Finally, the reflected THz is detected using a Schottky barrier diode (SBD). The dependency of the reflectance in sub-THz band on glucose and albumin concentrations in aqueous solutions has been measured in this experiment. It is observed that the reflectance is directly proportional to the concentration of glucose in the blood sample. Hence, the difference in the blood sugar levels of a healthy and diabetic person can be identified using the reflectance THz-TDS measurement.

12.11.2 DETECTION OF TUMOR-CANCER INFECTED CELLS

The most common cause of death is due to the growth of tumor-cancer cells in the body. Although conventional screening techniques are available, early diagnosis through accurate measurements with several parametric analyses was lagging until the emergence of THz technologies. The THz spectroscopy and imaging with a robotic arm in our body serves as a powerful tool for *in-situ* measurements. In order to obtain a reliable and high-resolution image of a layer of skin, organ, tissues, veins, and the like, inside our body, the safest electromagnetic spectrum is THz radiation because of its non-ionizing nature. It can produce microscopic and macroscopic transmission and reflection imaging with a fair contrast between diseased and normal cells.

The Figure 12.18 shows an experimental setup of a THz imaging system under reflection geometry. In this setup, LT-GaAs based PCA illuminated by a Ti:Sapphire

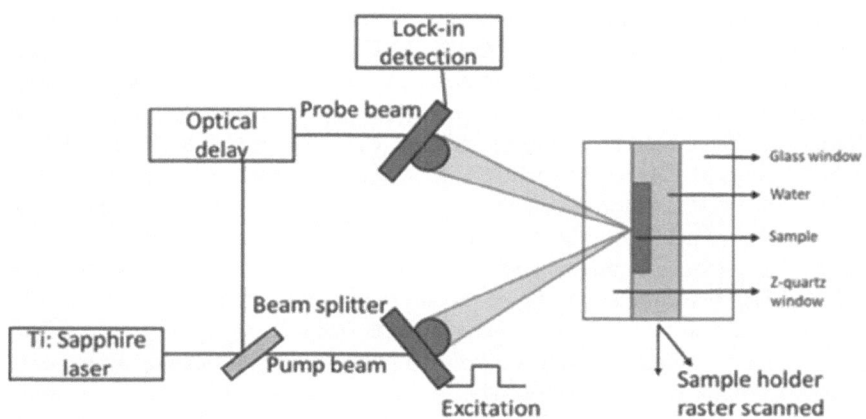

FIGURE 12.18 Experimental setup of THz imaging system under reflection geometry.

laser is used as a THz emitter and detector. The resulting THz radiation is focused through off-axis parabolic mirrors onto the sample and the reflected THz beam is collected at the detector in the presence of an optically chopped probe beam. The detection mechanism has already been described in section 12.3. The optical chopper has been used to sample the signal and the rapid scanning technique has been employed during THz imaging. The cuvette placed on a five-axis mount holds the sample for raster scanning. To maintain relative humidity of less than 10% during the experiment, nitrogen gas is purged in the path of the THz beam. The closed experiment setup is purged with nitrogen gas in-order to maintain the relative humidity of less than 10% and to make it free from atmospheric absorption.

The absorption and reflectance spectra of paraffin embedded tumor-cancer and healthy tissues can be observed in Figure 3 of Doradla et al. (2017) where the tumor assisted cancer cell has shown less absorption at 1.2 THz and 1.4 THz than the healthy cell spectra. This result shows the signature of other substances causing absorption rather than the water content.

The images of normal and tumor-cancer cells using digital photos as well as THz absorption and reflection can be visualized in Figure 4 of Doradla et al. (2017). The absorption figures (see Figure 3 [Doradla, Joseph, & Giles (2017)]) show more contrast between the healthy and tumor-cancer tissues than the figures from the reflection and optical images. Terahertz absorbance images and stained microanatomy images representing tumor-cancer and normal tissue can also be observed in Figure 10 of Doradla et al. (2017). It is noticeable that the THz absorption is higher for the tumor-cancer tissue than the healthy tissue.

Thus, these are a very few examples of THz applications in biomedical and healthcare systems. THz spectroscopy and imaging give accurate and reliable information in early-stage identification of infected areas.

12.12 CONCLUSION AND FUTURE ASPECTS

The common method to diagnose tumors is biopsy which is time-consuming and tedious. Magnetic resonance imaging and X-ray CT imaging are also used but these cause higher radiation doses. To detect cancer tissue in their early stages, terahertz technology can be efficiently used as it is non ionizing, has a short imaging time, and less radiation. The terahertz is very sensitive to water absorption between 0.04 THz and 0.8 THz, hence, it can easily identify infected tissues as human body has ~60% of water content. THz radiation is considered to be less harmful than X-rays and it also reduces the risk of heating tissue. However, these terahertz imaging technologies are facing some challenges in clinical application because of the lack of THz sources, and the lack of THz waveguides to reduce transmission losses in accessing the tissues. The interdigitated photoconductive antenna can be used as the efficient source to generate the terahertz radiation, and this makes the pulsed terahertz imaging system simpler due to its miniaturization and portability. This IPCA is micro and nano-structured which makes the device size small even at high frequencies with high efficiency and less loss. An antenna with high gain at terahertz frequency is required to proceed with further research on terahertz radiation in detecting tumor tissue, monitoring glucose level in patients, and so forth.

REFERENCES

Arnone, D. D., Ciesla, C. M., Corchia, A., Egusa, S., Pepper, M., Chamberlain, J. M., Bezant, C., Linfield, E. H., Clothier, R., and Khammo, N. Applications of terahertz (THz) technology to medical imaging. In *Terahertz Spectroscopy and Applications II* (pp. 209–219), vol. 3828. *International Society for Optics and Photonics*, 1999.

Arnone, D., Ciesla, C., and Pepper, M. Terahertz imaging comes into view. *Physics World*, 13(4), 35, 2000.

Auston, D. H., Cheung, K. P., and Smith, P. R. Picosecond photo conducting Hertzian dipoles. *Applied Physics Letters*, 45(3), 284–286, 1984.

Blaney, T. G. Signal-to-noise ratio and other characteristics of heterodyne radiation receivers. *Space Science Reviews*, 17(5), 691–702, 1975.

Boby, E., Prajapati, J., Rathinasamy, V., Mukherjee, S., and Mondal, S. Parametric Investigation of Interdigitated Photoconductive Antenna for Efficient Terahertz Applications. *Arabian Journal for Science and Engineering*, 47(3), 3597–3609, 2022.

Boby, E. N. F., Prajapati, J., Rathinasamy, V., Rao, T. R., and Mondal, S. 6G and beyond: Investigation of broadband terahertz interdigitated photoconductive antenna by exploiting laser parameters. *Microwave and Optical Technology Letters,* 64(12), 2197–2206, 2022.

Brun, M. A., Formanek, F., Yasuda, A., Sekine, M., Ando, N., and Eishii, Y. Terahertz imaging applied to cancer diagnosis. *Physics in Medicine & Biology*, 55(16), 4615, 2010.

Cai, Y., Brener, I., Lopata, J., Wynn, J., Pfeiffer, L., and Federici, J. Design and performance of singular electric field terahertz photo conducting antennas. *Applied Physics Letters*, 71(15), 2076–2078, 1997.

Crawley, D., Longbottom, C., Wallace, V. P., Cole, B., Arnone, D., and Pepper, M. Three-dimensional terahertz pulse imaging of dental tissue. *Journal of Biomedical Optics*, 8(2), 303–307, 2003.

Das, A. C., Bhattacharya, S., Mandal, K. C., Mondal, S., Jewariya, M., Ozaki, T., Bhaktha, S. N. B., and Datta, P. K. Dielectric response of pure and doped-GaSe crystals studied by an indigenously developed broadband THz-TDS system. In Benjamin J. Eggleton, Neil G. R. Broderick, and Alexander L. Gaeta (Eds.), *Nonlinear Optics and its Applications IV* (p. 98941E) vol. 9894. *International Society for Optics and Photonics*, 2016.

Doradla, P., Joseph, C., and Giles, R. H. Terahertz endoscopic imaging for colorectal cancer detection: Current status and future perspectives. *World Journal of Gastrointestinal Endoscopy*, 9(8), 346, 2017.

Elayan, H., Amin, O., Shihada, B., Shubair, R. M., and Alouini, M-S. Terahertz band: The last piece of RF spectrum puzzle for communication systems. *IEEE Open Journal of the Communications Society*, 1, 1–32, 2019.

Elayan, H., Amin, O., Shubair, R. M., and Alouini, M-S. Terahertz communication: The opportunities of wireless technology beyond 5g. In 2018 *International conference on advanced communication technologies and networking (CommNet)* (pp. 1–5), 2018.

El-Ghazaly, S. M., Joshi, R. P., and Grondin, R. O. Electromagnetic and transport considerations in sub picosecond photoconductive switch modelling. *IEEE Transactions on Microwave Theory and Techniques*, 38(5), 629–637, 1990.

Emadi, R., Safian, R., and Nezhad, A. Z. Investigation of saturation phenomena in spatially dispersive graphene-based photoconductive antennas using hot-carriers theory. *IEEE Journal of Quantum Electronics*, 53(5), 1–8, 2017.

Fathololoumi, S., Dupont, E., Chan, C., Wasilewski, Z., Laframboise, S., Ban, D., and Liu, H. Terahertz quantum cascade lasers operating up to 200 k with optimized oscillator strength and improved injection tunnelling. *Optics Express*, 20(4), 3866–3876, 2012.

Ferguson, B., and Zhang, X. C. Materials for terahertz science and technology. *Naturematerials*, *1*(1), 26–33, 2002.

Gadalla, M. N., Abdel-Rahman, M., and Shamim, A. Design, optimization, and fabrication of a 28.3 THz nano-rectenna for infrared detection and rectification. *Scientific Reports*, *4*(1), 1–9, 2014.

Geim, A. K., and Novoselov, K. S. The rise of graphene. In Peter Rodgers (Ed.), *Nanoscience and technology: A Collection of Reviews from Nature Journals* (pp. 11–19). World Scientific, 2010.

Godyak, V. A., Piejak, R. B., and Alexandrovich, B. M. Electrical characteristics of parallel plate rf discharges in argon. *IEEE Transactions on Plasma Science*, *19*(4), 660–676, 1991.

Gregory, I. S., Baker, C., Tribe, W. R., Evans, M. J., Beere, H. E., Linfield, E. H., Davies, A. G. and Missous, M. High resistivity annealed low-temperature GaAs with 100 fs lifetimes. *Applied Physics Letters*, *83*(20) 4199–4201, 2003.

Han, S-P., Ko, H., Kim, N., Ryu, H-C., Lee, C. W., Leem, Y. A., Lee, D., et al. "Optical fiber-coupled InGaAs-based terahertz time–domain spectroscopy system." *Optics letters*, *36*(16), 3094–3096, 2011.

Ji, Y. B., Lee, E. S., Kim, S-H., Son, J.-H., and Jeon, T-I. A miniaturized fiber-coupled terahertz endoscope system. *Optics express*, *17*(19), 17082–17087, 2009.

Kazemi, A. H., Mahani, F. F., and Mokhtari, A. Peak amplitude enhancement of photoconductive antenna using periodic nano slits and graphene in the THz band. *Optik*, *185*, 114–120, 2019.

Kenneth, K. O., Choi, W., Zhong, Q., Sharma, N., Zhang, Y., Han, R., Ahmad, Z., et al. Opening terahertz for everyday applications. *IEEE Communications Magazine*, *57*(8), 70–76, 2019.

Khiabani, N. Modelling, design and characterization of terahertz photoconductive antennas (Unpublished doctoral dissertation). University of Liverpool, 2013.

Khiabani, N., Huang, Y., Shen, Y-C., and Boyes, S. Theoretical modelling of a photoconductive antenna in a terahertz pulsed system. *IEEE Transactions on Antennas and Propagation*, *61*(4), 1538–1546, 2013.

Kim, K-Y. Generation of coherent terahertz radiation in ultrafast laser-gas interactions. *Physics of Plasmas*,*16*(5), 056706, 2009.

Krotkus, A., Marcinkevicius, S., Jasinski, J., Kaminska, M., Tan, H., and Jagadish, C. Picosecond carrier lifetime in GaAs implanted with high doses of as ions: An alternative material to low-temperature GaAs for optoelectronic applications. *Applied Physics Letters*, *66*(24), 3304–3306, 1995.

Lamarre, J-M., Désert, F-X., and Kirchner, T. Background limited infrared and submillimeter instruments. *Space Science Reviews*, *74*(1–2), 27–36, 1995.

Lee, K., Lee, S. C., Kim, W. T., Park, J., Min, B., and Rotermund, F. Terahertz generation by a resonant photoconductive antenna. *Current Optics and Photonics*, *4*(4), 373–379, 2020.

Lee, S-H., Choe, J-H., Kim, C., Bae, S., Kim, J-S., Park, Q-H., and Seo, M. Graphene assisted terahertz metamaterials for sensitive bio-sensing. *Sensors and Actuators B: Chemical*, *310*, 127841, 2020.

Lepeshov, S., Gorodetsky, A., Krasnok, A., Toropov, N., Vartanyan, T. A., Belov, P., Alú, A., and Rafailov, E. U. Boosting terahertz photoconductive antenna performance with optimized plasmonic nanostructures. *Scientific Reports*, *8*(1), 1–7, 2018.

Lepeshov, S. I., Gorodetsky, A. A., Toropov, N. A., Vartanyan, T. A., Rafailov, E. U., Krasnok, A. E., and Belov, P. A. Optimization of nanoantenna-enhanced terahertz emission from photoconductive antennas. *Journal of Physics: Conference Series*, *917*(6), 062060, 2017.

Liu, H., Yu, J., Huggard, P., and Alderman, B. A multichannel THz detector using integrated bow-tie antennas. *International Journal of Antennas and Propagation, 2013*, Article ID: 417108, https://doi.org/10.1155/2013/417108, 2013.

Liu, S., Zhang, C., Hu, M., Chen, X., Zhang, P., Gong, S., and Zhong, R. Coherent and tunable terahertz radiation from graphene surface plasmon polaritons excited by an electron beam. *Applied Physics Letters*, 104 (20), 201104, 2014.

Prajapati, J., Bharadwaj, M., Chatterjee, A., and Bhattacharjee, R. Circuit modeling and performance analysis of photoconductive antenna. *Optics Communications*, *394*, 69–79, 2017.

Rathinasamy, V., Thipparaju, R. R., Boby, E., and Mondal, S. Numerical investigation and circuit analysis of interdigitated photoconductive antenna for terahertz applications. *Optical and Quantum Electronics*, *54*(4), 1–18, 2022.

Rathinasamy, V., Thipparaju, R. R., Edwin, N. F. B., and Mondal, S. Interdigitated photoconductive terahertz antenna for future wireless communications. *Microwave and Optical Technology Letters*, *64*(12), 2189–2196, 2021.

Index

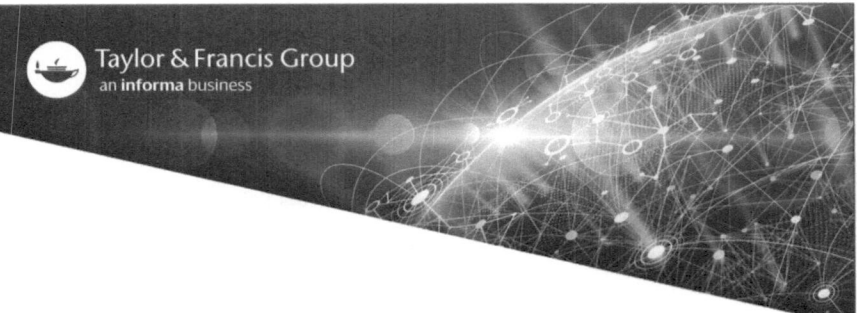
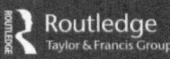
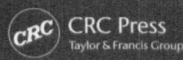